Understanding the Lingo

Check out the Glossary in Appendix A for a more complete list of menopausal terms. However, the following five terms should help you to understand the basics.

- **HRT (hormone replacement therapy):** A treatment to supplement the hormones you lose during menopause – generally a combination of oestrogen, progesterone, and sometimes testosterone.
- **Menopause:** Technically, menopause begins a year after your last menstrual period. Women whose ovaries are removed go through an immediate 'surgical menopause'.
- **Oestrogen:** This hormone is responsible for your female characteristics, such as breasts, curvy body, menstruation, and reproduction. The three types of oestrogen are: oestrone, oestradiol, and oestriol. Oestradiol, produced in the ovaries, is the most potent form of oestrogen and serves hundreds of bodily functions.
- **Perimenopause:** The years before menopause when your hormones are in flux and your periods are irregular. Some women are perimenopausal for up to 10 years before their periods actually stop, but normally the symptoms last only 4 or 5 years.
- **Progesterone:** A hormone that's made in larger amounts after you ovulate and release an egg. Progesterone is also produced in the placenta when you're pregnant to help prepare the uterus to nourish a fertilised egg. Synthetic forms of progesterone are called *progestogens.*

Symptoms that Say 'Menopause is Near'

Most women begin experiencing menopause symptoms, which are the result of hormones getting out of balance, while they're still having periods. If you experience several or all of the following symptoms, check with your doctor – you may be approaching the change.

- Dry skin or hair
- Fuzzy thinking (difficulty concentrating)
- Heart flutters (rapid heartbeats)
- Hot flushes
- Insomnia or interrupted sleep
- Irregular periods
- Irritability
- Memory lapses
- Mood swings
- Urinary problems (frequent urination or incontinence)
- Vaginal dryness

For Dummies: Bestselling Book Series for Beginners

The Five-Step Programme for Getting Through Menopause

Some women breeze through menopause without realising it's upon them, but others aren't so lucky. Here are a few ways to make the journey easier:

- Recognise that menopause is a natural transition, just like puberty. Fortunately, with a few more years under your belt, you are in a better position to ride out the storm of hormonal upheavals this time. Realise that menopause is a time of change, not only with your body but also with your life.

- Make sure that you have good two-way communication with your doctor – that means that your doctor listens to you, you listen to him or her, and that you feel comfortable with your doctor's advice.

- Re-evaluate your lifestyle. Your body is less forgiving now and lets you know if you continue with those bad habits you enjoy. You need to eat healthily, exercise regularly (at least five times a week), and get enough sleep. Maintaining a healthy weight helps you avoid a variety of serious medical conditions.

- Ask your doctor for a regular gynaecology examination and general check-up. Track any symptoms that you experience (both physical and mental) and discuss these with your doctor.

- Have patience with yourself. Find a way to relax and reduce your stress. Stress intensifies many menopausal symptoms and lowers your body's immunity to disease. Take time out for yourself to visit friends, join a yoga class, go for a walk, or do voluntary charity work – just anything that makes you feel good about yourself.

Flushing Out Hot Flushes

Because many women only start thinking about menopause when they start getting hot flushes, here's a few quick tips for dealing with hot flushes:

- Exercise regularly: Only one in 20 women who exercise regularly experiences hot flushes. Of women who don't exercise, one in four experiences hot flushes.

- Avoid caffeine and alcohol and watch those spicy foods and hot drinks. These can trigger hot flushes at the dinner table.

- Reduce your stress level by exercising or practising relaxation techniques.

- Layers are in – dress in layers so that you can peel off when you're flushing and cover back up when the flush has gone.

- Turn on a fan or throw the duvet back at night to avoid waking up with night sweats. Or switch to a sheet with several thin blankets so that you can adjust your layers when you need to.

For Dummies: Bestselling Book Series for Beginners

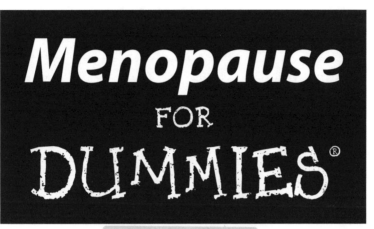

Menopause
FOR
DUMMIES®

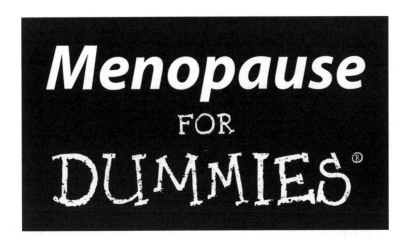

Menopause FOR DUMMIES®

by Dr Sarah Brewer, Marcia L. Jones, PhD, and
Dr Theresa Eichenwald

BICENTENNIAL
1807
WILEY
2007
BICENTENNIAL

John Wiley & Sons, Ltd

Menopause For Dummies®

Published by
John Wiley & Sons, Ltd
The Atrium
Southern Gate
Chichester
West Sussex
PO19 8SQ
England

E-mail (for orders and customer service enquires): cs-books@wiley.co.uk

Visit our Home Page on www.wiley.com

For general information on our other products and services, please contact our Customer Care
Department within the U.S. at 800-762-2974, outside the U.S. at 317-572-3993, or fax 317-572-4002.

For technical support, please visit www.wiley.com/techsupport.

Wiley also publishes its books in a variety of electronic formats.
not be available in electronic books.

British Library Cataloguing in Publication Data: A catalogue reco
British Library

ISBN: 978-0-470-06100-8

Printed and bound in Great Britain by Bell & Bain Ltd., Glasgow

10 9 8 7 6 5 4 3 2 1

About the Authors

Dr Sarah Brewer qualified as a doctor in 1983 from Cambridge University. She was a full-time GP for five years and now works in nutritional medicine and sexual health. Sarah is currently completing an MSc in Nutritional Medicine at the University of Surrey, Guildford.

Although her first love is medicine, her major passion is writing. Sarah writes widely on all aspects of health and has written over 40 popular self-help books. She is a regular contributor to a number of newspapers and women's magazines, and appears regularly on TV and radio. She was voted Health Journalist of the Year 2002.

Marcia L. Jones, PhD, had life experience in fertility treatment, perimenopause, and menopause. In 1991, while attempting to start a family at the age of 38, she scoured bookstores searching for down-to-earth information on the likely problems and how to proceed. Her doctor directed her to the only information available at the time, photocopies of technical articles from medical journals and pamphlets written by pharmaceutical companies trying to sell product. Today, many women are delaying childbirth, so the issue of fertility fits nicely into a discussion of perimenopause and menopause. These experiences served as her primary motivation for writing this book. She became certain that women in their mid-thirties to late forties need current, unbiased, reliable information on perimenopause and menopause written for a layperson.

Thanks to the efforts of her doctor, Jane Chihal, MD, a contributor to this book and a recognised expert on menopause and fertility, Dr Jones became the proud mother of two girls.

Dr Jones received her PhD from Southern Methodist University in anthropology. She led many research expeditions in the Middle East and served as an associate professor of anthropology at the University of Tulsa.

Growing weary of academia, Marcia shifted her career focus and entered the fast-paced world of software, achieving the rank of chief operating officer and co-owner of Criterion, a company that developed human-resource software for Fortune 1000 organizations. She grew Criterion from a $1.5 million company to a $10 million company and recently sold it to Peopleclick. Over the past 18 years, she wrote many articles on people in the workforce and taught courses in the use of human-resource technology as an adjunct professor in the Graduate School of Management at the University of Dallas.

Dr Theresa Eichenwald has extensive experience caring for menopausal women as an internist at hospitals in New York, Washington D.C., Philadelphia, and, most recently, Texas. She has taught at Albert Einstein School of Medicine and Mount Sinai Medical Center in New York.

In addition to teaching and caring for patients, Dr Eichenwald has authored a number of articles for professional journals, covering topics such as breast cancer and ovarian tumours as, well as patient education pamphlets. She is a member of the American Medical Association, the American College of Physicians, and in medical school participated in the American Medical Student Association Task Force on Aging.

Authors' Acknowledgements

From Sarah: I'd like to thank Marcia L. Jones and Theresa Eichenwald, authors of the original US version of *Menopause For Dummies*. The quality of their original script made my job easy, as I had so very little to do when adapting their excellent book for the UK market.

From Marcia: I am so grateful to the many talented people who have helped create this book. Special thanks to Dr Theresa Eichenwald for her contributions, collaborations, and review of early versions of this document. Thanks also to her husband Kurt Eichenwald and their three young sons for letting Theresa take the time to author this book.

Acknowledgement is due the Cooper Institute in Dallas for their continuing contributions in the field of preventative medicine.

Thanks to my women friends who insisted that this book was not only needed, but long overdue.

This book would never have gotten to Wiley Publishing if not for Richard and Ginger Simon.

Publisher's Acknowledgements

We're proud of this book; please send us your comments through our Dummies online registration form located at www.dummies.com/register/.

Some of the people who helped bring this book to market include the following:

Acquisitions, Editorial, and Media Development

Development Editor: Simon Bell

Commissioning Editor: Samantha Clapp

Developer: Colette Holden

Copy Editor: Kim Vernon

Proofreader: Lesley Green

Content Editor: Steve Edwards

Executive Editor: Jason Dunne

Executive Project Editor: Martin Tribe

Cover Photo: Getty Images/David Lees

Cartoons: Ed McLachlan

Composition Services

Project Coordinator: Jennifer Theriot

Layout and Graphics: Claudia Bell, Joyce Haughey, Stephanie D. Jumper, Laura Pence

Proofreaders: David Faust

Indexer: Aptara

Special Help

Brand Reviewer: Janet Sims

Publishing and Editorial for Consumer Dummies

Diane Graves Steele, Vice President and Publisher, Consumer Dummies

Joyce Pepple, Acquisitions Director, Consumer Dummies

Kristin A. Cocks, Product Development Director, Consumer Dummies

Michael Spring, Vice President and Publisher, Travel

Kelly Regan, Editorial Director, Travel

Publishing for Technology Dummies

Andy Cummings, Vice President and Publisher, Dummies Technology/General User

Composition Services

Gerry Fahey, Vice President of Production Services

Debbie Stailey, Director of Composition Services

Contents at a Glance

Table of Contents

Introduction

*W*e wrote this book to give women of all ages a clear view of the physical, mental, and emotional changes related to menopause. For generations, women of all ages have wandered blindly into menopause without knowing what to expect. Oh, you probably knew that menopause and hot flushes went hand in hand, but even that information isn't always true. The truth is that you may never have a hot flush, and if you do, it will probably be years before you're menopausal. Common knowledge about menopause is sparse and often wrong. (The medical community didn't even officially recognise the link between oestrogen and hot flushes until 1974!)

If menopause only concerned a small group of people on a desert island, this lack of information might be understandable. But over half of the world's population will become menopausal one day. Menopause has been the ugly family member of the research community for years. Even medical textbooks pay scant attention to the topic. Today, one group is paying attention to menopause. The pharmaceutical industry sees great opportunity in the field of menopause, and more research is under way. If you're looking for books to help reasonably intelligent women navigate the jungle of menopause (menopause is uncharted territory), your options are largely limited to pretty, glossy pamphlets published by drug companies (now that's what we call unbiased information) that you can find at your doctor's surgery. If you're really persistent, you may find some academic articles in medical journals, but your eyes will glass over as you try to pick out straightforward answers to your practical questions. We hope this book can fill that void. Our goal is to help you digest the research so you can make better and objective health decisions.

Menopause is not a disease – that's true. No one is going to die from menopause or its symptoms, but every day, women die from the medical effects of low oestrogen levels. Your risks of certain diseases and cancers rise after menopause. Some people may respond to that statement with one of their own, 'Well, that's because women are older when they go through menopause.' True again, but it's also true that oestrogen plays a role in an amazing number of functions in your body, some of which protect your organs, increase your immunity, and slow degeneration. This transformation we call menopause impacts our health in very significant ways. This book helps you understand the story behind the symptoms and the diseases.

Some women choose to use hormone therapy to relieve symptoms associated with menopause and protect their body from disease. The choice of whether to take hormones or not is quite controversial because hormone therapy has its own set of risks. The debate goes on in the medical community and media concerning the risks of hormone therapy. If you're like many women, your confusion only grows as you read more on the subject. Each new study seems to contradict the findings of the last one. You're an intelligent person. But how can you know which study you should believe? In this book, we try to provide enough information to enable you to make informed decisions about your health.

About This Book

We have no agenda in writing this book. We're not trying to sell you medications, alternative health strategies, or remedies. This book presents accurate and up-to-date information from the most credible sources. It contains straightforward information based on reliable medical studies without the academic lingo common to medical journals. When no clear-cut answers exist and when quality research shows mixed conclusions, we let you know.

Everyone's time is limited, so we cut to the chase. We cover the questions that are important to you during this phase of your life. If you want more detail, we provide an appendix full of resources to help with your personal research. We also try not to stray too far from the topic at hand. For example, during the years leading up to menopause, women may have difficulty getting pregnant. The same hormonal changes that cause those annoying symptoms prior to menopause also stifle fertility. Many women in their late thirties who are trying to get pregnant rely on hormone supplements. Despite the overlap in hormonal terms, fertility is not a concern for many women going through the change, so our discussion is limited.

Whether you're going through the change, have already been there, or are about to start off down that road, you'll find the information you need between these snazzy yellow and black covers. We cover all the health issues and therapy choices that confront women during the menopausal years.

Foolish Assumptions

Every author has to make a few assumptions about her audience, and we've made a few assumptions about you:

✔ You're a woman. (Sorry, guys, but menopause is a girls-only club.)

✔ You want to understand what's going on with your body.

✔ You're looking for straight talk for real people as opposed to scientific jargon and Medicalese (though we have a Medicalese icon to warn you when we stray into this territory).

✔ You want to evaluate your risks of disease as you pass through midlife and move into your menopausal years.

✔ You don't want a book that claims to let you diagnose yourself or figure out what medications you need. You have a medical advisor to discuss these things with.

✔ You want to be able to ask intelligent questions and discuss treatment alternatives with your healthcare providers.

✔ You want to feel more confident about the quality of your healthcare.

✔ You buy every book that has a black and yellow cover.

If any of these statements apply to you, you're in the right place.

How This Book Is Organised

We've organised this book into five parts so you can go directly to the topic that interests you the most. Here's a brief overview of each part:

Part I: The Main Facts about Menopause

The journey to menopause often catches women by surprise. You may not have been expecting to take the journey, or you may have been wondering when you would begin. In this part, we give you a quick overview of what your hormones are doing before, during, and after menopause. If you haven't thought about things like hormones and follicles for a while, don't worry; we refresh your memory. Your secondary school biology course probably never finished the story. In this part, you get the whole story from how the egg makes its journey from the ovary to the uterus to what happens when the ovary goes into retirement.

Part II: The Effects of Menopause on Your Body and Mind

Want to know how hormones affect the health of your body and mind? You can find the answers in Part II. We devote each chapter in this part to a specific body part or health issue. In each chapter, you get an overview of how hormones function in relation to this part of your body and the types of conditions that can develop, how to recognise them, and what you can do about them.

Part III: Treating the Effects

You may want to evaluate the pros and cons of hormone therapy (HT) from time to time during your journey through menopause. This part of the book brings you up to date on what the medical community knows about HT. We discuss the effects of HT so that you can make informed decisions. Reading these chapters provides added benefits as well: You'll probably find it easier to evaluate the news about hormone research that comes out in future years.

We also include information about non-HT drugs and alternative treatments.

Part IV: Lifestyle Issues for Menopause and Beyond

Part IV is chock full of great ways to stay healthy and enjoy a long and active life during and after menopause. Staying healthy and active is simpler than you think. We discuss healthy eating habits and simple ways to stay fit. Whether you're looking for natural ways to lower your risk of specific diseases or for ways to slow the ageing process, you can find the information you need right here.

Part V: The Part of Tens

If you're a fan of *For Dummies* books, you probably recognise this part. These are short chapters with quick tips and fast facts. In Part V, we debunk (more than) ten menopause myths, review some common medical tests you may encounter, and suggest ten terrific exercise programs for menopausal women.

Part VI: The Appendixes

A glossary of menopause-related terms and a list of menopause-related resources cap the book.

Conventions Used in This Book

We use our own brand of shorthand for some frequently used terms, and icons to highlight specific information. The following sections help you get used to these conventions.

Taking in shorthand

As you read this book, you'll discover that menopause is a process, with different stages characterised by similar symptoms. These stages are referred to as *perimenopause,* the 3 to 10 years prior to menopause when you may experience symptoms; *menopause* itself, which you know you've reached only after you've reached it because the definition of menopause is the absence of periods for a year; and *postmenopause,* which is your life after you've stopped having periods. In this book, we use *perimenopause* to describe the premenopause condition, and we use *menopause* to refer to everything after that just because the term *postmenopause* isn't commonly used.

A major part of this book – the whole of Part III as well as sections in other chapters – talks about hormone therapy (HT), which is used to alleviate symptoms and address health concerns prompted by menopause. In literature and on Web sites, you can see hormone therapies referred to and abbreviated any number of ways, including hormone replacement therapy (HRT) and estrogen replacement therapy (ERT). But we stick pretty closely to using HT because we feel that it's the most inclusive and accurate term. Just be aware that *HT* means essentially the same thing as *HRT.*

And, speaking of hormones, a couple of the more important ones for menopausal women have several subcategories:

- ✔ Types of **oestrogen** include oestriol, oestradiol, and oestrone.
- ✔ **Progesterone** is the class of hormone; the form used in hormone therapy is often referred to as progestin.

We sometimes use these terms interchangeably and only refer to the specific hormone as necessary for clarity.

Eyeing the icons

In this book, we use icons as a quick way to go directly to the information you need. Look for the icons in the margin that point out specific types of information. Here's what the icons we use in this book mean.

The Tip icon points out practical, concise information that can help you take better care of yourself.

This icon points you to medical terms and jargon that can help you understand what you read or hear from professionals and enable you to ask your healthcare provider intelligent questions.

This fine piece of art flags information that's worth noting.

When you see this icon, do what it tells you to do. It accompanies info that should be discussed with an expert in the field.

The Technical Stuff icon points out material that generally can be classified as dry as a bone. Although we think that the information is interesting, it's not vital to your understanding of the issue. Skip it if you so desire.

This icon cautions you about potential problems or threats to your health.

Where to Go from Here

For Dummies books are designed so that you can dip in anywhere that looks interesting and get the information you need. This is a reference book, so don't feel like you have to read an entire chapter (or even an entire section for that matter). You won't miss anything by skipping around. So, find what interests you and jump on in!

Part I
The Main Facts about Menopause

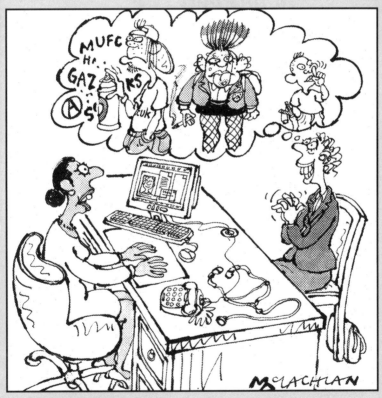

'Of course you realise the menopause
is the cessation of menstruation and signifies
the inability to have any more children.'

In this part . . .

The first act of *Dance of the Hormones* probably occurred three decades or so ago for you. You remember that one don't you? The bittersweet tale of teenage angst and joy that we call puberty. And now, intermission (the menstrual years) may be coming to a close as the hormones once again take the stage for the second act – menopause. Well, take your seat and get ready to peruse your programme . . . well, Part I of this book, anyway.

In Part I, we provide you with an outline to your menopausal years. We define menopause, review the biology, introduce you to the actors – your hormones – and briefly review the related symptoms and health conditions (physical, mental, and emotional). Get to it before the usher dims the lights.

Chapter 1

Reversing Puberty

In This Chapter

▶ Getting your feet wet with the basics on menopause

▶ Figuring out where you are on the menopausal road map

▶ Understanding the symptoms of menopause

▶ Outlining the healthcare options for a long and healthy life

*'Y*ou've come a long way, baby' is a recurring slogan for baby boomers. The phrase certainly says a lot about women in this generation as they approach that rite of passage known as menopause. As an individual, you no doubt feel you've come a long way too, as your menopause approaches. Society, in general, and women, in particular, have also come a long way in opening up full and frank discussions about the mysteries of menopause.

Puberty and menopause bracket the reproductive phase of your life. They have a lot in common: They're both transitions (meaning that they don't last forever), they're both triggered by hormones, and they both cause physical and emotional changes that can make you feel like you're going a little crazy.

The beginning of your reproductive years. Remember the journey? Your hormone levels shifted wildly and caused your first menstrual period. And don't forget the erratic emotions that are the hallmark of teenage angst. But over the course of a few years, your hormones found a comfortable level and righted themselves again. Your unpredictable periods finally settled into a predictable pattern, and your emotional balance was more or less restored.

At the end of your reproductive years, your hormone levels go through a similar journey, this time causing the mid-life crisis, but your hormones eventually find a new, lower level of production. Your periods are erratic for a while, but they eventually wind down and stop. And just in case you're wondering, those mid-life emotional crises eventually pass, too.

Keep in mind that the phrase 'You've come a long way, baby' closes with 'but you've still got a long way to go'. Women today often live 40 or 50 years after the menopause. Most of us want to enjoy these years by visiting friends, taking care of our loved ones and ourselves, and continuing to participate in activities that give us pleasure.

In this chapter, we introduce you to the menopause so that you know what to expect when the time comes, or explain what is happening if the transition is already here.

Defining Menopause

Do you ever notice how you don't really pay close attention to where you're going when you're the passenger in a car? You only start to worry about exit junctions and traffic lights when you're the one behind the wheel. Well, menopause is just like that. We all hear about menopause and menopausal symptoms, but we rarely pay attention to the particulars until our turn arrives.

When you do slide into the driver's seat and start paying attention, you may become frustrated by the confusing terminology associated with the whole menopause thing. Aside from the pamphlets you get from your doctor's surgery, most books, magazines, and articles treat menopause like a stage that starts with hot flushes and goes on for the rest of your life. But, *menopause* actually means the end of menstruation. During the years leading up to menopause (called *perimenopause*), your periods are often so erratic that you're never sure whether *this* period is the last one, but you aren't officially menopausal until you haven't had a period for a year.

A lot happens before you have your last period, and all this physical and mental commotion is associated with menopause. You may experience hot flushes, mental lapses, mood swings, and heart palpitations while you're still having periods. But, when you ask your doctor whether you're menopausal, he or she may check you over and say no. Relax: Your doctor isn't wrong, and you aren't crazy. You're not menopausal. You're *peri*menopausal.

Medical folks divide menopause into phases that coincide with physiological changes. We describe these phases later in this chapter, but you need to know something about the terminology that surrounds menopause. On the one hand, you have the medical terms associated with menopause, and on the other, you have the terms that you hear when you're chatting with your friends.

The term *perimenopause* refers to the time leading up to the cessation of menstruation, when oestrogen production slows down. A lot of the symptoms that folks usually label as *menopausal* (hot flushes, mood swings, sleeplessness, and so on) actually take place during the perimenopausal years. This book is a stickler about using the term *perimenopause* rather than *menopause* to describe this early phase because you're still having periods. We also use *perimenopause* to underline the physiological and emotional changes you experience before the end of your periods, which helps to distinguish these changes from those that happen after your body starts adjusting to lower levels of oestrogen.

Technically, the time after your last period is called *postmenopause,* but this word has never really caught on. So, in keeping with common usage, we most often use the term *menopause* to refer to the actual event and the years after menopause and use the more clumsy term *postmenopause* only when it helps to clarify things. When we talk in this book about *menopausal* women, we mean women whose periods have stopped – whether they're 55, 75, or 105 years old.

The years leading up to and following menopause mark a pretty major transformation in your life. As you make your way through this phase, you probably want to know where you're at within the whole grand scope of the change and what's going on inside you. Here's a brief description of the phases associated with menopause. (Don't worry: Other chapters give you a lot more detail about the various stages.)

Making changes while approaching the change: Perimenopause

Perimenopause is the stage when your hormones keep changing gear. Some months, your hormones operate at the levels they've worked at for the past 30 years or so; other months, your ovaries are tired and don't produce as much oestrogen as they should. Your brain responds to this lack of oestrogen by sending a signal to try to jump-start those ovaries. Then, when they receive the signal, your ovaries leap into action and overcompensate for their laziness by producing double or even three times as much oestrogen as they should.

Your period may be late because your ovaries were dozing during the first part of your normal cycle. Then, when your period does come, it may be super heavy because, when your ovaries wake up, they overcompensate by producing much too much oestrogen.

So, during perimenopause, you still have your period, but you experience symptoms that people associate with menopause. If you go to the doctor at this stage and ask, 'What's happening to me? Is this the menopause?', the doctor often goes straight to the 'Is this the menopause?' part of your question and says, 'No, of course you're not menopausal if you're still having periods.' But many doctors miss the first part of your question – the 'What's happening to me?' part. This is the real issue to which you want an answer – the cause of your weird physical and emotional experiences that make you feel like everything's going haywire.

Menstruating no more: To menopause and beyond

Menopause means never having to say, 'May I use one of your tampons?' again.

Women usually become menopausal some time between the ages of 45 and 55 years, with an average age of 51, though the age is getting later and later. New research suggests that every year, the average age of menopause increases by one month. At whatever age it happens, if you haven't had a period for one year, you've reached *menopause*. This definition may seem cut and dry at first glance, but here are a few situations that may leave you scratching your head:

What if you use a cyclical type of hormone therapy in which you take oestrogen for several days, and a progestin (synthetic form of progesterone hormone) during the last few days of your cycle? You still have a period (well, technically a 'hormone withdrawal bleed' as stopping the progestin causes you to shed the lining of the uterus), but you don't ovulate. Are you menopausal or not? Technically, you're delaying your last period. You're taking a sufficient dosage of oestrogen to rid yourself of perimenopausal symptoms, but you're no longer fertile.

Here's another tricky one: If you've had a *hysterectomy* (surgical removal of the uterus), you're menopausal according to the basic definition. But, if your uterus is removed but your ovaries are left in place, you're not 'hormonally' menopausal because your ovaries still produce oestrogen. By doing blood tests to analyse your hormone levels, your doctor can tell you whether or not your hormones are officially at menopausal levels.

These tricky situations may lead you to ask, 'Who cares about the definition?' You know a rose is a rose. The main concern here is *what's happening with your hormones*, especially oestrogen. Hormonal changes can trigger many physical and emotional health issues.

When you reach menopause, your hormone production is so low that your periods stop. Your ovaries still produce some oestrogen, progesterone, even testosterone, but instead of producing hormones in cycles (which is why you have periods and why you're only fertile for about four or five days each month), your body now produces constant, low levels of hormones. The type of oestrogen your ovaries churn out also switches from an active type to a rather inactive form.

Postmenopause is the period of your life that starts after menopause (a year after your last period) and ends when you do. Postmenopause is a time when your body produces greatly reduced levels of oestrogen, testosterone, and progesterone. In this book, we refer to both the cessation of your period and your life afterwards as . . . menopause.

Anticipating Menopause

When can you expect the menopause? The timing varies from woman to woman. Predicting this stuff is nowhere near an exact science. You can't even use the fact that you started your period earlier than most women as a predictor that you'll stop menstruating earlier. The same goes for starting your period later in life and ending it later in life. In fact, modern women both start their periods earlier and finish them later than they did just a generation ago. Genetics, lifestyle (especially smoking), and nutrition have some impact on the schedule, but basically menopause just happens when it happens. But we can give you average age ranges for these phases.

Most women become perimenopausal some time between the ages of 35 and 50 years. You'll probably know when you get there because you have some of the symptoms (check out the Cheat Sheet at the front of this book and Chapter 3 for more on the symptoms of menopause) and/or some irregular periods. Women usually become menopausal some time in their fifties.

Some events can alter these 'normal' age patterns, including lifestyle habits and medical interventions. Here are a few exceptional types of menopause:

- **Premature menopause:** This is a term for when women go through menopause in their thirties or earlier. This timing is considered unusually early.
- **Medical menopause:** This refers to menopause due to chemotherapy or radiation therapy. Sometimes these treatments cause a temporary pause in your body's normal cycle, so this type of menopause often reverses after treatment is finished, though your periods may take a month, several months, or even years to return.

✔ **Surgical menopause:** This refers to menopause due to surgery. Removal of the womb and both ovaries results in an immediate, non-reversible menopause.

Because your ovaries produce all types of sex hormones (oestrogen, progesterone, and testosterone), surgical removal of your ovaries is fairly traumatic for your system, and you typically experience intense perimenopausal symptoms (hot flushes and the like).

Excessive exercising or an eating disorder can cause a temporary halt in your periods (a condition called *amenorrhoea,* which means 'absence of menstruation'), but your periods will probably return to normal when your lifestyle returns to normal. Such a situation is not menopause but rather a medical condition that needs treatment.

Experiencing Menopause

When a group of women talk about their personal experiences of puberty, menstrual cycles, and pregnancy, the stories are all different. Some women don't notice changes in their bodies; others recognise the moment ovulation or even conception occurs. Some women have terrible problems with pre-menstrual syndrome (PMS); others have trouble-free cycles throughout their entire lives. Women's experiences vary with perimenopause and menopause just as much as they vary with these other changes.

Men-o-pause

When men experience mood swings and mental lapses during their fifties, they (or you) may think that they're going through the change, too. But the change men go through is quite different from the one women experience.

The rise and fall of hormones in a woman's body follows a cyclical pattern. Hormone levels shift throughout the month on a regular basis. So, every 28–35 days, a woman has the chance to become pregnant. The hormonal changes prepare her body for conception and pregnancy.

Men have no cycle – apart, perhaps, from the yearly sporting calendar. Their primary sex hormone, testosterone, stays at a fairly constant level from day to day, so men don't experience cyclical fluctuations. But men's testosterone levels do decline with age. Lower testosterone levels generally result in lower libido (sex drive) in males and generally occur when men are in their late fifties or sixties.

Do men go through menopause? There's no question that the decline of sex hormones in men results in lower libido, weaker bones, and an increased risk of prostate cancer. But the changes are simply a result of the natural ageing process and are not triggered by a change in hormonal patterns.

Identifying symptoms

Chapter 3 describes the various symptoms women may experience during the perimenopausal years. Chapters 10 through 14 explain the link between your hormones and how hormone replacement therapy (HRT) can help these symptoms.

Less than half of all women experience annoying symptoms such as hot flushes, heart palpitations, interrupted sleep, and mood swings during the transition period before menopause. Most women who do experience these symptoms experience them while they're still menstruating on a regular schedule.

Other women recognise that they're perimenopausal because their periods change from being regular as clockwork, to being irregular and totally unpredictable. Their periods may come late or early, they may skip a period, or their flow may be light one month and resemble a flood the next.

Unfortunately no medical test can determine whether you're officially perimenopausal or not.

Calling in the professionals

If you're in your late forties or fifties and you're experiencing the symptoms listed on the Cheat Sheet and in Chapter 3, you can probably assume that you're perimenopausal. But don't cancel that appointment with your doctor to get things checked out (and if you don't have an appointment to cancel, make one and keep it). Many symptoms of perimenopause are the same as some of the symptoms of thyroid problems, cardiovascular disease, depression, and other serious health issues.

Your medical practitioner can help you deal with the undesirable symptoms of perimenopause and prevent the serious health conditions that are more prevalent after menopause.

Making Time for Menopause

You may wonder when the perimenopause and menopause phase of your life will hit and how long the symptoms will last.

Starting out

Most women's ovaries begin a transformation some time between the ages of 35 and 50. If you start the change before you reach 40, you experience what's known as *premature menopause*.

Perimenopause is sometimes called a climacteric period, which simply means a crucial period. Remember that your ovaries don't just shut down one day; the transition is punctuated with production peaks and valleys that may cause many annoying physical and mental symptoms. Perimenopause is a time of important physiological changes – and the time when egg production starts to slow along with the production of oestrogen and progesterone.

Seeing it through to the end

Because you never really know when perimenopause starts, accurately defining a timeframe is difficult. Some women experience symptoms for ten years before their periods stop. Most of the symptoms you hear about are due to the fluctuating hormone levels of perimenopause rather than the sustained, low levels of hormones you experience during menopause.

You're officially menopausal one year after your last period. After that, many people use the term postmenopause to mark the rest of your life (though this book just keeps using the term *menopause*).

Treating Menopause

At the end of the perimenopause road, your ovaries (and consequently, your hormone production) finally wind down. Your body gradually adjusts to the lower hormone levels typical of menopausal life. Most of the perimenopausal symptoms disappear, but now your concerns shift to health issues associated with prolonged, lowered levels of active oestrogen.

Oestrogen not only plays a role in reproduction: It also helps to regulate a host of other functions throughout your body. Oestrogen protects your bones and cardiovascular system, among other responsibilities. Those pesky perimenopausal symptoms may make life miserable, but they aren't dangerous to your health. However, the conditions associated with long periods of diminished oestrogen levels are both troublesome and potentially harmful. They include

- ✔ Coronary heart disease
- ✔ Hypertension (high blood pressure)
- ✔ Osteoporosis
- ✔ Stroke

We suggest that you and your doctor work together on strategies to prevent these conditions from happening.

Some women choose hormone replacement therapy (HRT) to help prevent disease; others choose to take medications as individual problems arise. (We cover hormone therapy in Chapters 10–15 and non-hormonal ways to deal with certain conditions in Chapter 17.) Some women prefer to take a more natural route and rely on alternatives to traditional medicine such as herbs, homeopathy, and acupuncture to see them through (check out Chapter 16 for more on complementary medicine). Whichever path or paths you choose, each strategy has benefits and risks. Your choices depend on your medical history, your family history, and your healthcare preferences. And remember that both your experiences and medical technologies change daily, so re-evaluate your options from time to time.

Promoting Longevity

Not so long ago, 50 years was about as old as we expected to live. Today, many of us can expect to live well into our seventies, eighties, nineties, and beyond. The fact that most women are no longer fertile after their forties doesn't mean that women are no longer productive after this age. In fact, with the whole reproduction thing out of the way, women have more time and opportunities to make new contributions to life on earth (or in space!).

One of the keys to a long and happy life is choosing your parents carefully so you inherit good, healthy genes that encourage longevity. Another key is taking good care of yourself and the genes you're dealt. Regular check-ups can address many medical issues as they arise and help prevent other conditions from developing. In addition, eating healthy foods (and portions) and taking lots of exercise can help you live life to its fullest.

Most people agree that a healthy lifestyle is the best way to reduce troublesome perimenopausal symptoms, prevent disease, and promote a long and healthy lifespan. Following a healthy lifestyle is also the least risky strategy for dealing with perimenopause and menopause. Taking up the challenge of adopting a healthy lifestyle requires self-assessment and a bit of determination. Shifting to a healthy lifestyle involves eliminating unhealthy habits, getting at least half an hour of aerobic exercise five times a week, and maintaining a healthy, balanced diet that includes at least five (and preferably more) servings of fruit and vegetables each day. Chapters 18 and 19 provide lots of info on diet, nutrition, and exercise to keep you right on track.

Chapter 2

Talking Biology and Psychology: Your Mind and Body During Menopause

*I*f you're in your forties, and you're like a lot of women, you may have asked yourself 'What in the world is happening to me?' Perhaps it's those stray hairs on your chin that are starting to resemble eyebrows, or that persistent ring of fat around your waist that brings the question to mind. You know what we're talking about – that extra girth that seemingly appears overnight and won't go away no matter how many sit-ups you do. Or maybe you notice yourself perspiring in bed, just like you did when you first got together with your partner – except now it happens in the middle of the night when you're not even thinking about *that*. Does it seem as if the world is getting dumber and no one can do anything right anymore? Maybe it's not the new millennium that's causing your irritability and mood swings: Maybe you're hitting perimenopause.

This chapter takes a look at how your hormones work during your reproductive years and how they change as you approach and enter your nonreproductive phase. The physiological, emotional, and mental changes you may notice during perimenopause and menopause are largely triggered by fluctuations or deviations in your hormone levels.

Setting the Stage

Menopause is a natural and necessary change in life. Menopause isn't a disease, deficiency, or failure. You may read medical terms such as o*estrogen deficiency*, *ovarian failure*, and *vaginal atrophy* (or thinning) but these terms aren't meant to carry negative connotations. They're meant to describe expected conditions. Viewing menopause as a natural change – not an organ failure – is important.

Just as women aren't put on the earth for the single purpose of bearing children, so your ovaries aren't there only to supply eggs. Your ovaries live a double life – one as the holder of the seeds of life (*oocytes*, which later develop into eggs), and the other as a factory maintenance worker. Menopause marks the shift from the first life to the second life. No longer busy with developing follicles that both carry eggs and release lots of oestrogen, your ovaries move on to the methodical production of low levels of hormones to maintain body functions.

Your ovaries are a critical source of hormones for your body and continue to produce hormones well after menopause, but in much smaller amounts than before. Your ovaries don't retire; they just experience a career change and take things a little easier. They deserve it.

Because the life expectancy for most women in Great Britain is about 80 years, the average female spends around half her life menstruating and perhaps using contraception to control her fertility. Therefore, you can expect to spend a significant portion of your later life just being a woman – not going through puberty or menopause or the periods in between.

Medical professionals who view menopause as a natural change focus less on trying to 'fix a failure' and more on future health issues.

Making the Menstrual Cycle and Hormone Connection

Okay, admit it. You didn't pay much attention to those long, boring, biology lessons explaining menstruation during school. Or the educational films with titles like 'Now You're a Woman'. (Back in those days, interesting titles like *Sex For Dummies* didn't exist.) If you were anything like us, you had difficulty making a connection between the two-dimensional, black-and-white illustrations of female bits and the three-dimensional, high-definition experiences of bloating and cramps.

Days of our lives: Determining day 1

The first day of your period is called day 1. Simple enough, eh? Sounds pretty obvious. Well, maybe not. When it comes to your body, nothing is ever truly definitive. Here's how things can get complicated: Do you count yesterday as day 1 because you had light bleeding? Or do you call today day 1 because you really started flowing today? Or maybe you should count two days ago as day 1 because you

started cramping really badly and had a bit of spotting.

How to solve this dilemma? Consistency is key. If you normally have a light day before your regular flow starts, count your light day as day 1. But, if you experience spotting several days before your period actually starts, then count day 1 as the first day of your regular flow.

In this section, we, hopefully, make the connection between your sex hormones and your lifelong menstrual cycle in a clearer, more meaningful fashion than your dear old biology teacher made it.

One of the main functions of your sex hormones is to prepare your body to produce life. So viewing your sex hormones as they work together as a team is a good place to start the discussion. Then we take a closer look at each individual member of the hormone team.

The average menstrual cycle is 28 days, but a cycle that lasts anywhere from 22 to 35 days is normal. For the purpose of this discussion, we use a 28-day cycle; you can adjust the numbers as necessary to fit your personal calendar. Figure 2-1 shows hormone levels throughout a menstrual cycle.

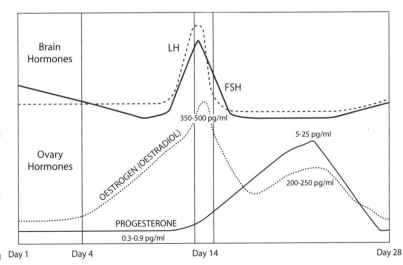

Figure 2-1: Hormone levels throughout the menstrual cycle.

Day 1 of your cycle is the first day of your period (see the sidebar 'Days of our lives: Determining day 1' for help determining the first day of your period). Your body begins flushing out the lining of your uterus, which isn't needed because a fertilised egg requiring nourishment and support isn't present in your uterus.

Your ovaries are filled with little seeds (eggs) surrounded by support cells (*stroma*). During the first half of your cycle (days 1 to 14), hormones produced in your brain – *follicle-stimulating hormone* (FSH) and *luteinising hormone* (LH) – and hormones produced in your ovaries – oestradiol, oestrone and oestriol – together known as oestrogen work together to develop and then release an egg. (For more on FSH and LH, see 'Heading up your hormones' later in this chapter.) During these first two weeks, your oestrogen levels are on the rise, and your progesterone levels are very low. This particular hormone combination (high oestrogen, low progesterone) is why you usually feel so good during this stretch of your cycle. You owe your energy, restful sleep, upbeat mood, sharp memory, and terrific concentration to your old friend, oestrogen, which plays a role in many physical and mental systems – not just your reproductive system.

As soon as your brain senses that oestrogen levels are right, it produces a surge of LH, which triggers the release of an egg – otherwise known as *ovulation*. Ovulation usually occurs between days 12 and 16 of your cycle. (For the scoop on LH, check out 'Heading up your hormones' later in this chapter.)

After ovulation, oestrogen levels drop, and progesterone production kicks in. *Progesterone*, which peaks around day 20, is a hormone that gets the uterus ready for a baby. If the egg is fertilised, your progesterone levels stay high. If the egg isn't fertilised, progesterone and oestrogen levels drop and menstruation occurs.

Surveying the Role of Hormones

Unless you're a gynaecologist, you don't need to remember what all the hormones do or what their abbreviations stand for. So here's Table 2-1 as a quick review of the most important hormones and their functions.

Table 2-1		Hormones in a Nutshell
Hormone	*Produced By*	*Main Activities*
Oestrogens	Ovaries	Female hormones that promote breast development and play a big role in menstrual cycles, ovulation, pregnancy, and more.

Hormone	Produced By	Main Activities
Oestrone (E1)		An 'inactive' form of oestrogen. After menopause, oestrone is the dominant form of oestrogen in your body. Oestrone is produced in the ovaries before menopause. After menopause, body fat produces oestrone. High levels of oestrone are linked with breast and endometrial cancer.
Oestradiol (E2)		The 'active' form of oestrogen produced mainly in the ovaries. Services hundreds of mental and physical functions in a woman's body. Before menopause, oestradiol is the dominant form of oestrogen in your body.
Oestriol (E3)		Form of oestrogen found mainly in pregnant women.
Follicle-stimulating hormone (FSH)	Pituitary gland	Hormone produced in the brain that stimulates the ovaries to get follicles growing and producing oestrogen. This is the hormone FSH that kicks off the ovulation cycle.
Luteinising hormone (LH)	Pituitary gland	Hormone produced in the brain that triggers the follicle to release the egg (ovulation). LH supports the production of oestrogen and progesterone by the abandoned empty egg sac known as the *corpus luteum.*
Progesterone	Ovaries	Prepares the womb for pregnancy and helps maintain pregnancy. Oestrogen is the dominant hormone in the first half of your menstrual cycle, but progesterone is dominant in the second half. The effects of progesterone also include water retention, sweet sugar cravings, and fatigue. High doses of progesterone can work as a sedative or as a depressant. The synthetic forms of progesterone are called *progestins.*
Testosterone	Ovaries	Considered a 'male hormone' even though the bodies of both men and women produce it. In women, the ovaries produce testosterone, and so, during the menopause, testosterone levels drop. Testosterone benefits women by maintaining healthy libido, strong bones, and muscle growth.

Heading up your hormones

Your brain produces the hormones that direct the production of sex hormones in your ovaries. Think of the hormones produced in your brain as senior management, directing operations in your ovaries, whose hormones are the field managers, directing operations in the field, which is your entire body. The hormones made in your brain include:

- **Follicle-stimulating hormone (FSH):** When your brain senses that oestrogen and progesterone levels have dropped, it shoots out FSH to tell the ovaries to begin developing *follicles* (nutritious sacs that cover the eggs) and start producing oestrogen.

- **Luteinising hormone (LH):** This hormone triggers ovulation. When LH surges, the follicle releases the egg. The abandoned follicle wrapping, the *corpus luteum,* secretes both progesterone and oestrogen.

Explaining oestrogen

Oh, how sophisticated women are! We don't just produce oestrogen. We produce three different types of oestrogen:

- **Oestradiol:** Active oestrogen

- **Oestrone:** Inactive oestrogen, which is predominant after the menopause

- **Oestriol:** Oestrogen produced mainly during pregnancy

In this book we use the generic term *oestrogen* to mean all the different types of oestrogen, unless distinguishing among them is particularly important (and it hardly ever is).

Oestradiol

You may hear doctors and nurses refer to oestradiol by its scientific name, *17-beta oestradiol,* but most people know it as 'the good stuff'. Before menopause, oestradiol is the predominant form of oestrogen produced in your ovaries and used throughout your body. Oestradiol actively helps out with hundreds of different physical and mental functions.

After menopause, your ovaries stop producing oestradiol, and that's when you develop many of those annoying symptoms such as hot flushes, palpitations, changes in your skin, aching joints, dry hair, headaches, and so on.

Your body can convert oestrone to oestradiol but only if your ovaries are fully functioning. Your ovaries slow down during perimenopause and menopause and your body doesn't get nearly as much oestradiol after menopause as it used to during your reproductive years.

Oestrone

After menopause, oestrone is the predominant type of oestrogen streaming through your body. Oestrone is made by your body fat and, before menopause, in your ovaries, too. The more body fat you have, the more oestrone you have. Oestrone is mainly a stored form of oestrogen. Before menopause, your ovaries can convert oestrone to the active form of oestrogen, oestradiol, but this conversion only happens in premenopausal ovaries.

Oestriol

The weakest of the three oestrogens is oestriol, which is produced mainly in the placenta during pregnancy. When you are not pregnant, the amount of oestriol in your body is small – similar to that found in men, actually. Oestriol is also used in certain brands of hormone replacement therapy (HRT).

Promoting progesterone

If all these hormone names are confusing, here's a tip to help make sense of progesterone. Think of progesterone as *pro*moting *gest*ation: Progesterone prepares your womb to nurture a fertilised egg.

Most progesterone is made after ovulation. If your egg is fertilised, the placenta takes over progesterone production during the eighth or ninth week of pregnancy. If the egg isn't fertilised, progesterone levels drop. It is this lack of progesterone that triggers your period. Many doctors believe that symptoms of premenstrual syndrome (PMS) are due to changing levels of progesterone. You can thank progesterone when you crave sweets, feel fatigued, retain water, develop acne, have a premenstrual emotional melt-down or feel bloated.

Why? Well, progesterone is designed to get your body ready to support a pregnancy. So, when progesterone levels are high, you feel hungry more often. Progesterone also slows down the digestion process so that you can absorb nutrients better, but that slower digestion process can make you feel bloated or constipated.

Progesterone can also cause depression and has a sedating effect that makes some women feel calm and others feel lethargic. Such things are all a matter of perception, but the sedating effect isn't just your imagination.

Investigating androgens

Yes, your body does produce 'male' hormones – this is perfectly normal and even desirable. Both men and (to a lesser degree) women produce a group of hormones called androgens in their adrenal glands and sex organs (testes in men, ovaries in women). The androgens affected at the menopause are testosterone and DHEA (whose meaning is explained a bit later in this section).

As you get older, your body slows its production of both female and male hormones. During perimenopause, oestrogen and androgen levels can get out of balance. Even though your androgen levels typically decrease as oestrogen levels decrease, the big fall in oestrogen levels can alter the balance so that androgen has a greater relative presence than it did before menopause. This imbalance leads to rather annoying changes:

- Fat migrates towards your waist.
- Hair disappears from your head and starts growing on your chin and upper lip.
- Your blood pressure rises.
- Your cholesterol level rises.

But you can stop cursing now. All the news is not bad, as androgens also have many positive effects for women:

- **Testosterone:** This hormone triggers sexual desire. That's right – testosterone promotes a healthy sexual appetite in women. Testosterone also helps women build bone, maintain muscle mass (so you burn fat), and maintain optimal energy levels.
- **DHEA:** *DHEA* stands for *dehydroepiandrosterone*. DHEA is a building block for testosterone. Your ovaries convert DHEA (from your adrenal glands) into testosterone. Without DHEA, you can forget about all those positives associated with testosterone.

DHEA is not available in pharmacies in the UK but is advertised on the Internet. Don't be tempted to buy DHEA as it can cause unwanted side effects if you're not careful. For DHEA to work, you need functioning ovaries and the presence of oestradiol – but during perimenopause and beyond, your ovaries aren't peak performers and your oestradiol level drops. Because the sale of DHEA is unregulated, you may not know how much you need or how much you're getting.

Acting Out the Stages of Menopause

Menopause, the permanent pause in your periods (*menses*), is one of those things that you aren't sure has happened until long after it's over. Like the first time you met your current best friend: You probably had no idea you'd become so close and you only realise how special that occasion really was when you look back on it now. Okay, so menopause isn't exactly a warm and fuzzy card occasion, but is, nevertheless, a passage worth noting.

Are you or aren't you menopausal? You can answer that question only after you've enjoyed a year without your period. Many of the annoying symptoms assigned to menopause actually are much worse before menopause in the phase known as *perimenopause*. During perimenopause, you get both the annoying symptoms (hot flushes, irritability, mood swings, and so on) and your period. Lucky you!

In this section, we clarify what happens to your body during the various stages of menopause and explain how to recognise where you are in the great transition.

Previewing perimenopause

For most women, perimenopause is a big case of *déjà vu*. Remember puberty? The crying spells? The mood swings? The 'What's wrong with my skin?' traumas? Well, guess what? They're back! Once again, your hormones are ready to wreak havoc on your body, your emotions, and your mental faculties. This time around, however, you're a bit wiser (you bought this book, didn't you?), you have experience dealing with change, and you realise that this phase too shall pass.

Some doctors (usually male) advise women who are still experiencing periods not to worry about 'menopausal' symptoms. But you know (because you read it here) that you feel the symptoms often attributed to menopause as intensely or more intensely during perimenopause. And perimenopause can last for ten years before you stop menstruating altogether and become truly menopausal.

Periodic periods

During perimenopause, things change. If you have welcomed your period on the same day as the full moon for 20 years, you may wake up to find the planets are suddenly out of alignment.

The hormonal shift is due to earthquake-like upheavals in your ovaries. Your ovaries hold little *oocytes* (seeds), and each month some of these seeds develop into *follicles* (little sacs that hold an egg). One or two lucky follicles mature and release an egg. That's when you ovulate. The oocytes in your ovaries are held together by a substance called *stroma*. The stroma produces testosterone, and the follicles produce oestrogen. Between birth and puberty, you have hundreds of thousands of these little seeds with only a little stroma in-between. As you get older, you have fewer seeds and relatively more stroma. As the mix of seeds and stroma in your ovaries changes, so does hormone production. Your ovaries decrease their production of oestrogen but continue to produce testosterone.

During perimenopause, sometimes you ovulate during your cycle; sometimes you don't. Sometimes the FSH just doesn't tickle up your remaining follicles as well as usual, so oestrogen levels are low at the beginning of your cycle instead of high. Your brain responds to this lack of get-up-and-go by sending another surge of FSH (see 'Heading up your hormones' earlier in this chapter for more on FSH). Finally getting the message, your ovaries become a little frantic and go into double-time production of oestrogen. Right at the time when you should be ovulating and producing progesterone, your ovaries are just kicking into gear developing a follicle. That means you don't ovulate when you usually do and your period is late (and heavy).

Your menstrual cycle is all messed up. Your oestrogen level shoots up, and then it drops down. You may get hot flushes and heart palpitations (racing heart) when your oestrogen level plunges. And just when you're convinced that something is funny and you need to schedule a doctor's appointment, you get your period and everything returns to normal. You wonder why you were so worried and cancel the doctor's appointment – until the next weird thing happens.

All the above is perfectly fine (maybe not with you, but with Mother Nature) – it's all part of perimenopause.

Emotional emotions

For some women, it's not the disrupted sleep, hot flushes, or palpitations that get their attention – it's the mood swings which mean you leap from happy to sad, or experience anxiety and panic attacks for no apparent reason. In contrast, other women find they no longer have to cope with pre-menstrual syndrome (PMS) and actually feel more emotionally stable than before. While it's easy to blame emotional changes on falling hormone levels, this time of life is also one where you can encounter other stresses such as caring for elderly relatives, offspring leaving home and a husband in the full-throes of a mid-life crisis. If your mood swings are pronounced, it helps to take an energetic form of exercise such as a brisk walk or even a jog. Exercise releases brain chemicals such as endorphins that help to lift your mood and keep you on a more even keel. Welcome to perimenopause!

Mental fog

You may be familiar with the roles your hormones play in your mental agility and emotional stability during your menstrual cycles and, perhaps, pregnancy. When your oestrogen levels drop and progesterone levels rise before your period, you get those annoying PMS symptoms such as fuzzy thinking, mood swings, fatigue, and restless sleep.

As your hormone levels jump around during perimenopause, these annoying symptoms are common. Oestrogen is involved in managing a number of brain operations, and when oestrogen levels take a dive during perimenopause, you can feel like you're guiding a boat that periodically loses its rudder. Here are a few of the mental functions that oestrogen helps to manage – and a few of the symptoms you experience when oestrogen takes a dive:

✔ Serotonin production. *Serotonin* regulates sleep, pain, libido (the posh word for sex drive), mood, and other mental functions. Less oestrogen means more problems in all these areas.

✔ Body-temperature control. You may experience hot flushes and night sweats.

✔ Pain threshold. You may be more sensitive or intolerant to pain.

✔ Attention, mental focus, and concentration. You may have mental lapses.

✔ Communication between nerve cells related to memory. You may become forgetful.

Meeting menopause

The onset of menopause, according to the medical definition, takes place a year after your last period. Few medical conditions use an anniversary date as a basis for diagnosis, but menopause is one of the few. That's why figuring out who's in the club and who's not is so hard. After menopause, you're technically *postmenopausal* for the rest of your life. The term *postmenopausal* hasn't really caught on in common usage, and so in this book we use the term *menopause* to mean both menopause and your postmenopausal years.

As far as your body is concerned, reaching menopause is almost a non-event. Your ovaries have slowed down over several years, producing lower and lower levels of oestrogen and releasing eggs only sporadically.

Most of the symptoms ascribed to menopause generally begin during peri-menopause. But back-to-back years of lower oestrogen-production can result in health issues that you don't notice until menopause sets in properly. Over time, lower levels of oestrogen (oestradiol in particular) can contribute to osteoporosis (brittle bones), coronary heart disease, stroke, and other diseases. Due to these possible complications later in life, your doctor may start measuring your height and keeping a closer eye on your cholesterol levels, blood pressure, and lifestyle habits (like exercise and diet) as you approach mid-life.

Menopause is the time to review your diet, exercise routine, and unhealthy habits (smoking or excessive consumption of alcohol, for example). In your earlier life, your body was forgiving. During menopause, it won't let you get away with unhealthy habits. During menopause, gaining weight is easier, and losing it harder, than when you were younger. And getting a good night's sleep and waking up feeling refreshed and ready to take on the day isn't as easy as before. Make healthy resolutions and stick with them so that you don't wind up saying, like composer Eubie Blake, when he turned 100, 'If I'd known I was going to live this long, I'd have taken better care of myself.'

Prepping for Surgical Menopause

Total removal of your ovaries is a shock to your body. If a surgeon removes both your ovaries during a gynaecological operation, you immediately go into menopause. This process is called *surgical menopause*. Instead of the gradual transition through perimenopause into menopause, you pop the oestrogen clutch and go spinning downhill into menopause. Your hormone levels drop instantaneously, except for those produced in the adrenal gland – testosterone and oestrone.

To save you from a sudden complete absence of hormones, your doctor may suggest you take hormone replacement therapy (HRT) to allow your body to make the transition more smoothly to the new state of affairs. If you've had your ovaries removed, take note: Some experts believe you're at greater risk of osteoporosis and heart disease. (Check out Chapters 4 and 5, respectively, for more on these conditions.)

If you have only one ovary removed, you may go through a normal, natural menopause if the other ovary continues to work properly. One ovary can produce enough eggs for a pregnancy, and enough hormones to keep your body in good shape, assuming you aren't approaching menopause anyway.

A *hysterectomy* (removal of your uterus) technically shouldn't slow down your ovaries' production of hormones. You will probably still go through a natural menopause because your ovaries are still intact and producing hormones. Women who have had a hysterectomy often go through menopause one to three years earlier than women who have not had a hysterectomy, possibly because surgery ties off and reduces some of the blood vessels (arteries) supplying blood to the ovaries, which go on strike and shut down earlier than normal as a result.

Menopause is defined as reaching the one-year anniversary of your last period. But your uterus is gone, and so you don't have periods. How do you know when you clear that hurdle? The only way to know is by watching the other symptoms – the restless-sleep habits, hot flushes, heart palpitations, and so on, and on. If you experience the classic perimenopausal symptoms, you're probably entering perimenopause and your hormones are rising up and sinking low. You're probably menopausal when your symptoms settle down.

Chapter 3

Getting in Sync with the Symptoms

*Y*ou're irritable for no reason, you have trouble sleeping, you experience heart palpitations, and your sex drive is dwindling. Sound familiar? If so, you're almost certainly starting down the road to menopause.

Every human body is unique, but the path to menopause reveals just how different we really are. Some women breeze through the change, experiencing few physical or emotional indications that anything is happening. Other women experience disturbing symptoms for an extended period of time. Fortunately, the symptoms usually pass as you move into menopause and beyond.

In this chapter we introduce you to the perimenopausal and menopausal symptoms you may experience. We go into greater detail concerning the biology of menopause in Chapters 4 to 9, and how to alleviate these symptoms Chapters 10 to 17.

Although the symptoms we discuss in this chapter are all symptoms of perimenopause and menopause, they're not *unique* to perimenopause and menopause. Other medical conditions can cause these symptoms as well. If you experience any of these symptoms, don't just assume they're a result of your changing hormones: We suggest that you see your doctor to check out other possible causes.

Kicking Things Off with Perimenopausal Symptoms

In this section, we describe the symptoms that are attributed to the sudden drop in oestrogen levels during perimenopause. You may experience none, a few, or a lot of these symptoms to a greater or lesser degree. If this sounds wishy-washy, then hands up, we're guilty as charged: In this book we hedge our bets because each woman is unique.

If you are yet to experience perimenopause or menopause, take heart in the following statistic – but if you are currently experiencing symptoms you may want to hide the following fact from the folks you live with – only 40 to 60 per cent of women in the western world report experiencing any perimenopausal symptoms. For women who do experience symptoms, these range in severity from somewhat annoying (think of an inability to find your favourite chocolate brand in your local shop) to interfering with their ability to enjoy life (think of your favourite chocolate company going out of business!).

Getting physical

When you heard Olivia Newton-John belt out 'Let's get physical' a million years ago, did you ever think it would come down to this? Well it has, so here's an outline of the physical side of perimenopause – as in the outward, physical signs that your body's hormones are a-changing.

Many of the physical symptoms are the result of a string of events that happen when *oestradiol* (the active form of oestrogen – refer to Chapter 2) levels drop suddenly – a typical occurrence during perimenopause. The drop causes a chain reaction in your body; for more on this, see the sidebar 'Revealing the biology behind the symptoms' later in this chapter.

Although researchers don't have all the details yet, they do know that oestrogen plays some kind of role in the production and maintenance of serotonin, a brain chemical that helps your body regulate sleep and moods. This relationship between oestrogen and serotonin plays a role in many of the mental symptoms of menopause and also has a hand in some of the physical symptoms, such as difficulty with sleeping.

Turning up the heat

Hot flushes are the traditional, highly recognised symptom of menopause. When you have a hot flush, you suddenly feel flushed – especially in your face and upper body. Increased perspiration usually accompanies this feeling of warmth. You may also have dizziness, heart palpitations, and a suffocating feeling.

A sudden drop in oestrogen levels triggers a hot flush. This drop in oestrogen sends a message to your brain that something is terribly wrong, so your brain sends out a power burst of adrenaline (epinephrine). *Adrenaline* is the hormone that triggers the fight-or-flight response in humans, so your body moves into ready mode, which gets your blood pressure up and your heart pounding and causes the blood vessels in your head, neck, and chest to dilate. All this commotion makes you feel like you're sweltering.

Until 1970, doctors didn't recognise hot flushes as a real physical phenomenon: They attributed the sensation to a woman's imagination or to a psychological problem.

Sweating your lack of sleep

Night sweats are essentially hot flushes that occur at night. The same oestrogen drop that triggers hot flushes during the day triggers night sweats.

Night sweats can also mean you have an infection, thyroid problem, or another illness. If night sweats are your only seemingly perimenopausal symptom, check with your doctor.

Losing your snoozing time

With all these weird symptoms going on during the day, getting a good night's sleep so you can wake up feeling rested doesn't seem like a lot to ask for, but sleep is often a big problem. Hot flushes in the middle of the night can easily interrupt your sleep. You wake up, often perspiring and sometimes cursing, and have a hard time dropping off to sleep again. Interrupted sleep can cause sleep deprivation, which in turn leads to irritability, anxiety, and mood swings.

A rapid drop in oestrogen also affects your serotonin level, which, in turn, helps regulate mood and sleep patterns. (Antidepressant drugs such as fluoxetine and sertraline work on the principle that serotonin regulation is key to relieving mood swings, irritability, and so on.) Oestrogen makes serotonin more available by prolonging the action of serotonin. A drop in your oestrogen level affects your serotonin levels, which contributes to interrupted sleep patterns.

Getting to the heart of the palpitation issue

Butterflies in your stomach often accompany heart flutters, or *palpitations*. The sudden drops in oestrogen that are so common during perimenopause cause reactions all over your body (more on this in the sidebar 'Revealing the biology behind the symptoms' later in this chapter), including heart flutters. The drop in oestrogen causes your body's natural painkillers and mood regulators (*endorphins*) to drop. Your body interprets this state of affairs as trouble, so a command is issued to send out a burst of adrenaline (epinephrine), the 'fight-or-flight hormone'. You respond as though you've just encountered a big grizzly bear. The only trouble is you don't see the grizzly bear, and you're left wondering why your body suddenly decides to get ready to flee just as you sit down to a nice candle-lit dinner.

Expecting menstrual irregularities

The approaching menopause is to blame for a number of menstrual irregularities. But remember that you can't blame all irregularities on perimenopause. Although these menstrual symptoms often wait for women on the road to change, we suggest you consult your doctor about these and all other symptoms before simply writing them off as perimenopause.

- ✔ **Irregular periods** are quite common in perimenopausal women as fluctuating hormone levels interrupt the ovulation cycle. Some months you ovulate; some months you don't. If you don't ovulate, you don't produce enough progesterone to have a period, so the lining of your uterus continues to build up.

- ✔ **Heavy bleeding** during perimenopause is usually due to an 'eggless' cycle. You make oestrogen during the first part of your cycle, but for some reason (often unknown) you just don't ovulate. Therefore, you don't produce progesterone, and you develop an unusually thick uterine lining, which you shed during your period. This process translates into abnormally heavy bleeding.

- ✔ **Bad timing** has probably struck every woman at one point or another. Don't think that perimenopause is going to make dealing with your periods any easier. As long as you still have periods, they're liable to show up at inconvenient times – which makes getting rid of them sound like not a bad thing at all.

Handling the headaches

If you experience intense headaches during the first few days of your period, we have bad news – you may have more headaches during perimenopause. Headaches during the first few days of your period mean that you're sensitive to low oestrogen levels, which are typical at that time. When oestrogen levels drop quickly, which happens during perimenopause, the drop may trigger another one of those headaches.

TIP

Revealing the biology behind the symptoms

The symptoms of menopause are all tied to plunging hormone levels. You may feel these symptoms more frequently during perimenopause than menopause because your hormone levels fluctuate more during perimenopause. Sometimes they rise to fairly normal levels, and then they come crashing down. The fluctuation is the trigger for a lot of your symptoms. When you reach menopause, your hormone levels are consistently lower than during your reproductive years, so your hormones don't pop up and drop down so frequently as during perimenopause. As a result, many women find their symptoms actually improve once their periods stop, though symptoms can still occur.

Here's a step-by-step guide to what happens to your body when your levels of oestradiol (the active form of oestrogen, as we explain in Chapter 2) drop:

1. Your ovaries produce lower levels of oestradiol, which causes a drop in the amount of oestradiol reaching the brain.

2. Less oestradiol in your brain causes a decrease in your endorphin levels. *Endorphins* are your body's natural painkillers and mood regulators. (If you're a runner, you're probably familiar with the effects of endorphins – they cause the 'runner's high'.)

3. Lower levels of endorphins in your brain cause your brain to think that something is terribly wrong, so it sends out a burst of adrenaline, the hormone that triggers the fight-or-flight response.

4. The burst of adrenaline causes your body to kick into ready-for-anything mode by increasing your heart rate (which causes those palpitations and flutters), raising your blood pressure, and dilating (widening) your blood vessels. Those dilating blood vessels are responsible for your hot flushes and sweating. If you're asleep, you may wake up suddenly. You may also experience diarrhoea or get a feeling of anxiety and butterflies in your stomach.

Facing the fibroid factoids

Fibroids are balls of uterine muscle tissue, rather like knots in a piece of wood. Nearly a third of women have fibroids by the time they're 50 years old. Fibroids tend to get bigger as you approach menopause, but they usually don't grow in size after the menopause. Fibroids are often 'symptomless', but can cause enlarged tummy, painful periods and heavy periods.

You don't need to do anything about fibroids unless they cause symptoms such as pain, pressure, or increased bleeding. If you develop these symptoms, see your general practitioner who can arrange tests to confirm the diagnosis. Treatments include drugs to reduce bleeding and surgery to remove either the fibroids, the lining of the womb, or the womb itself (*hysterectomy*). The treatment of choice depends on the size and number of your fibroids, and whether or not your family is complete.

Playing head games

The mental and emotional symptoms associated with perimenopause are often frustrating, but many women don't associate their irritability or depression with perimenopause.

The emotional symptoms we list here generally pass after your hormones settle into their new, lower levels after menopause. However, these symptoms severely inconvenience or otherwise bother many women during perimenopause. If this description mirrors your situation, don't sit there suffering in silence.

Tell your doctor about your mental and emotional symptoms as they are usually related more closely to hormonal imbalances than to psychological issues. Your doctor or other healthcare practitioner can ensure that you get the proper treatment to alleviate your symptoms. (For more information on the mental and emotional issues associated with perimenopause, check out Chapter 9.)

Sitting on the mood swings

Mood swings are common in perimenopausal women. But remember that mood swings are also common before your period (part of premenstrual syndrome (PMS)) and after pregnancy. Although medical researchers don't know all the details, low levels of oestrogen are associated with lower levels of serotonin, which can lead to mood swings, as well as irritability, anxiety, pain sensitivity, eating disorders, and insomnia.

Worrying about anxiety

Anxiety is another common symptom that perimenopausal women face. Like mood swings, anxiety is tied to low levels of oestrogen, probably because low oestrogen levels are associated with lower levels of endorphins and serotonin. Another theory is that low levels of oestrogen, serotonin, and endorphins leave you more susceptible to the emotional stressors in your life. According to this theory, lower oestrogen, serotonin, and endorphin levels don't trigger anxiety: Those lower levels simply inhibit your ability to deal easily with stressful situations.

Touching on irritability

The same hormonal shifts that cause mood swings and anxiety also cause irritability. Like these other symptoms, irritability is a temporary condition that seems to blow over after you reach the menopause.

Recalling memory malfunctions

Memory problems during perimenopause sneak up on you. You forget your friend's name one day; you leave your keys somewhere the next. Soon, you start remembering how many times you couldn't remember something. We're not talking dementia or Alzheimer's disease here; we're describing forgetfulness and a lack of focus. This category covers relatively minor memory glitches: You forget what you're about to say mid-sentence, or you get to the shop and forget what you need to buy. Thank goodness for sticky notes and grocery lists.

Oestrogen seems to facilitate communication among *neurons* (nerve cells) in the brain. Much of memory is a matter of the brain sending information from one memory storage centre to another. Because oestrogen helps maintain and grow new connections, shifting oestrogen levels can stymie communication between memory storage zones. Although memory problems are often only a short-term issue, it's worth using a few tricks to improve your recall, such as writing notes to yourself on sticky pads and leaving them in obvious places.

Researchers still don't know whether hormones have anything to do with more permanent types of dementia and Alzheimer's disease. But studies suggest that oestrogen can reduce the risk, or at least slow down the progression, of Alzheimer's disease later in life.

Thinking through a haze

Fuzzy thinking is common when you're deprived of sleep and your hormones are in flux. By *fuzzy thinking*, we mean the feeling that you're just not with it today – like you're walking through a fog or you can't concentrate on what you're doing.

Fuzzy thinking can result from interrupted sleep, which isn't uncommon during perimenopause. Fluctuating hormone levels also cause fuzzy thinking, just like in pregnancy and at certain points in your menstrual cycle. Like many of the symptoms that accompany perimenopause, this too shall pass. Fuzzy thinking is a temporary thing and generally clears up when your hormones settle down and your sleep patterns chill out during menopause.

Meeting the Menopausal Symptoms

All the symptoms we describe as *perimenopausal* are usually attributed to menopause. But after you're menopausal (without a menstrual period for a year), things begin to settle down a bit. Your hot flushes should subside and your moods stabilise. Your body and psyche seem to get used to some aspects of lower oestrogen production.

The symptoms you experience after menopause, however, are sometimes a bit more uncomfortable physically.

Long periods of low levels of oestrogen encourage conditions such as osteoporosis, cardiovascular disease, heart attack, stroke, and colon cancer, (look at Chapters 4, 5 and 13 for more on these).

We use the term *menopause* in this book to refer to the time period that includes both menopause and postmenopause.

Figuring out the physical facts

After your ovaries retire (well, they never really retire – they just greatly reduce their workload), you produce lower levels of oestrogen without the sudden spikes and drops typical of perimenopause. Your hormones calm down – way down. As time goes by, these long periods of low oestrogen levels result in a few physical changes.

In this section we discuss what these conditions feel like. We go into greater detail about the biology behind these conditions and how to alleviate the symptoms in other chapters of this book. (Chapter 6 deals with vaginal and urinary issues; Chapter 7 covers your skin and hair during menopause.)

Some of your symptoms are the result of lower levels of oestrogen, pure and simple. We call these primary symptoms. Some of these primary symptoms can actually cause further unpleasantness, which we call secondary symptoms.

Peering at the primary symptoms

The primary symptoms include:

- **Hair changes:** Your hair becomes thinner and more brittle with menopause, though some women report that their hair feels as soft and fluffy as cotton several years into menopause. Oestrogen is a natural moisturiser, so with lower levels of the stuff flowing through your body, your hair takes a hit and becomes more brittle. You may also have a tougher time keeping a perm permanent.

- **Skin changes:** Lower oestrogen levels cause your skin to sag and wrinkle. Oestrogen doesn't literally prevent sagging, but oestrogen does keep your skin elastic and help your skin to retain fluid, so it remains 'filled out' rather than becoming loose and droopy.

✔ **Urinary frequency:** Like incontinence, urinary frequency results from sustained, low levels of oestrogen that define menopause. Urinary frequency simply means that you have to urinate frequently. You may leave the bathroom and quickly feel like you have to go again. This condition is frustrating during the day – and even more frustrating at night. Urinary frequency can also interrupt your sleep, which, understandably, may make you irritable.

✔ **Urinary incontinence:** This condition is much more prevalent in women after menopause than it is during the reproductive years. The tissues of your urinary tract become drier and thinner, and the muscles lose their tone as oestrogen levels diminish. You know you're experiencing urinary incontinence if you have to try hard not to wet yourself when you laugh, exercise, or sneeze. Your urinary tract, especially your urethra, depends on oestrogen to maintain its form and muscle tone. The urethra has a hard time sealing off the flow of urine after years of diminished oestrogen levels.

✔ **Vaginal dryness:** This is known medically as *vaginal atrophy*. Because oestrogen keeps your vaginal tissues moisturised and pliant, continuous periods of low oestrogen can result in the drying out and shrinking of your vaginal tissue. Between 20 and 45 per cent of women experience vaginal dryness, which is most noticeable when intercourse becomes painful due to a lack of lubrication.

✔ **Vulvar discomfort:** Itching, burning, and dryness of the vulva isn't uncommon among menopausal women. But remember that many conditions and diseases that affect your vulva have nothing to do with oestrogen, so ask your doctor to check out any vulvar changes.

✔ **Weight changes:** Your weight shifts to the centre of your body – around your waist. Instead of the pear-shaped body you once had, you take on more of an apple shape due to shifting hormone levels. Although you may gain a bit of weight, you probably can't blame that directly on hormonal changes: Your body simply becomes less forgiving about nutritional imbalances and poor eating, drinking, and exercise habits.

Sussing out the secondary conditions

The bad news is not over yet. One or more of the primary symptoms can trigger even more unpleasantness. Here you go:

✔ **Fatigue:** If you consistently don't get a good restful night's sleep or you experience insomnia, you may become fatigued. But fatigue can also result from low testosterone levels.

✔ **Interrupted sleep:** Hot flushes, urinary frequency, anxiety, and a variety of other menopausal symptoms can all interrupt sleep during the night.

You may wake up feeling tired and experience fatigue throughout the day because your body isn't able to enter the deep stages of sleep at night.

✔ **Painful intercourse:** Experiencing pain during intercourse is generally the result of vaginal dryness or physical changes in the position of the urethra; this is due to changes in the shape of the vagina that happen over time when oestrogen levels are continuously low. As low levels of oestrogen cause the tissues of the vagina and urinary tract to become thinner, and the supporting muscle to lose its tone, your organs naturally shift position a bit.

Discovering that menopause is more than skin deep

The mental and emotional aspects of perimenopause are more of a mixed bag. Some symptoms experienced during menopause usually decrease or go away completely; others are a bit more difficult to deal with.

✔ **Anxiety:** Often, the anxiety common during perimenopause is due to the rapid drop in oestrogen, which initiates a chain reaction (see the sidebar 'Revealing the biology behind the symptoms' earlier in this chapter). After menopause, unexplained anxiety often dies down and you return to your normal self.

✔ **Depression:** If you have had a hysterectomy, you're more likely to experience menopause-related depression than a woman who goes through a natural menopause. Researchers don't understand why this is so.

If you take oestrogen hormone replacement therapy and suddenly stop taking it, rather than going through a weaning process, you may have more problems with depression. Oestrogen assists in the production of serotonin (a substance which helps regulate moods), so lower levels of oestrogen can lead to lower levels of serotonin.

✔ **Headaches:** If you experience your first migraine during perimenopause, you will likely find the migraines go away after menopause.

✔ **Lower libido:** Decreased sex drive is a problem for many menopausal women, but the good news is that 70 per cent of women remain sexually active during their perimenopausal and menopausal years. Lower libido is linked with hormonal imbalances and may result when testosterone levels are too low. (For more information on menopause and your libido, take a look at Chapter 8.)

> ✔ **Memory lapses and fuzzy thinking:** Although memory lapses and fuzzy
> thinking are common during perimenopause, most women notice that
> their concentration and memory return to normal after menopause.
> Ageing can cause mental impairment later in life, but you can't blame
> everything on menopause!

Unravelling the Mystery of Menopause

Many people associate the word *symptom* with disease, but according to the
dictionary definition a symptom is a condition or event that accompanies
something else. Sometimes you only see perimenopause in your rear-view
mirror. You may not know that you are going through perimenopause until
years later.

For many women, perimenopausal symptoms surface at one time or another.
You may feel that weird things keep happening to your body or your emotions, but it may take a little investigation on your part to bring the whole
perimenopause into focus.

Maybe you feel a flutter in your chest and you're convinced you're on the
verge of a heart attack. If you see a cardiologist to check out your heart palpitations, the cardiologist probably won't even think to check your hormones
because he or she's looking for something in your heart to answer the riddle.

Or maybe the 'weird things' going on with you aren't physical at all. Maybe
they're emotional – such as becoming easily frustrated at work or shouting at
the kids 50 times a day for the last two weeks. Many women may think twice
about these symptoms but don't bring them up with their doctor. If you do
mention them to your doctor, he or she may say, 'It's nothing.' Nothing? We
can guess what you're thinking: 'Try telling that to my work colleagues and
my kids!'

After you get a hot flush or two, you may figure out that these 'weird things'
aren't part of your imagination and that you're getting close to menopause. If
you figure out the connection, consider yourself lucky. Few women realise
that the heart palpitations and irritability are part of the same condition –
perimenopause. As you're reading this book, you're now the local expert – it's
up to you to coach other women through this!

Even gynaecologists sometimes overlook a hormonal imbalance as the
source of symptoms. A woman may suspect that her problem is 'chemical' or
hormonal only to have a doctor say that she's too young for menopause or
that as she's still having periods she isn't menopausal.

Some gynaecologists go so far as to take a blood test to check your FSH (follicle stimulating hormone) level to rule out menopause. High levels of FSH are indicative of *menopause*. But during perimenopause, your hormone levels go up and down. One month your FSH is perfectly normal; another month it's high. Without getting tested month after month, determining whether you're *perimenopausal* is difficult.

But women's oestrogen and testosterone levels can (and usually do) get out of whack even before they officially become menopausal, and the imbalance triggers the annoying symptoms often associated with menopause. Sometimes seeking medical advice can be even more frustrating because the experts tell you 'It's nothing' or alarm you with the number and types of tests that they want you to take.

The reality is that the symptoms you experience are often more intense during perimenopause than they are after the change.

Part II
The Effects of Menopause on Your Body and Mind

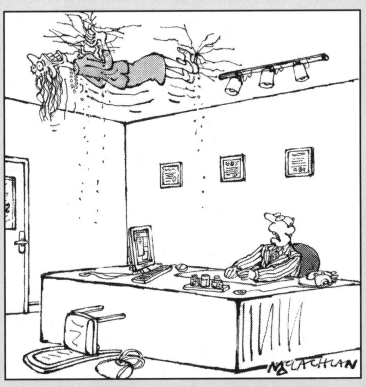

'This hypertension of yours – If I mention the word 'menopause' ....?'

In this part . . .

Are you convinced that the goldfish is deliberately trying to aggravate you? Has your family recently taken to wearing gloves and parkas in the house because you insist on turning the heating off? We jest because we've been there. But the years before and after menopause can bring a whole host of symptoms and conditions with them – from the simply annoying to the potentially dangerous. Don't worry: Knowledge is power! In this part, we cover the physical, mental, and emotional symptoms and conditions that women run into. We deal with your bones, cardiovascular system, reproductive organs, skin, hair, sex life, and mental and emotional outlook. Pretty thorough, huh?

Chapter 4

Boning Up on Your Bones

*M*ost women don't want to just live through menopause: They want to dance through it and keep dancing for another 40 or 50 years. Healthy bones keep your get-up-and-go from turning into sit-down-and-wait.

Osteoporosis literally means 'porous bone'. Osteoporosis is a disease, in which your bones become thin and fragile and more likely to break. In fact, osteoporotic bones in the spine may be so fragile that your own weight crushes them. When you pack apples on top of the soft bread in your shopping bag, the weight of the apples deforms the bread. A similar thing happens when the bones in your back press down on each other – you develop a so-called dowager's hump.

You can lower your risk of developing osteoporosis by building healthy bones before menopause and making healthy choices in your lifestyle after menopause.

Why are women more susceptible to osteoporosis after menopause? Why are women more prone to osteoporosis than men? What's the connection between oestrogen and osteoporosis? What can you do after menopause to save your bones? This chapter gives you the answers to these questions and shows you ways to help keep your bones dancing through the menopause and beyond.

Homing In on Bone Health

Knowing how your body makes bones and knowing how to keep them healthy is a good place to start when outlining the relationship between the change and the health of your bones. Your bones don't stop growing after you become an adult. They're alive and changing throughout your life.

Growing big bones and strong bones

When you're a kid, it's obvious that your bones are growing. As your bones get longer, you get taller. But your bones don't just grow longer; they also get thicker – denser. The denser your bone, the more difficult it is to break your bones. Think of a dinner service: Those thick earthenware plates you have at home are much more difficult to break than the fragile, translucent, fine china you see in expensive restaurants. People with strong bones have dense bones. Your bones continue to increase in density until you're about 30 years old, at which age you reach *peak bone density*. The ideal goal of all young women is to try to make their bones more like earthenware than fine china as they reach the age of 30. If you start building strong, dense bones when you're young, the effects of bone loss in mid-life tend to be less problematic. The higher your peak bone density, the better chance you have of keeping your bones healthy.

In the animal kingdom, males are usually bigger than females; men also tend to have denser bones than women. On average, black women have denser bones than white and Asian women. This is why men in general and black women tend to have less trouble with osteoporosis than white and Asian women.

Understanding peak bone density

Peak bone density is the maximum amount of bone that you'll ever have. Most people reach their peak around the age of 30. Maximising your peak bone density is important because, after the age of 35, you lose more bone than you build.

Your peak bone density depends on a number of factors such as genetics, diet, and exercise. You can't control your genes – you're born with them. Among other things, genes control the size of your frame and your ability to produce bone. But you can control your diet to get plenty of calcium, vitamin D, and magnesium, and you can exercise early in life so that you maximise your peak bone density. Avoiding alcohol and not smoking also helps you reach a high peak bone density.

TECHNICAL STUFF

Remodelling your house of bones

To better understand osteoporosis, it helps to look at how bone is 'built'. Each bone contains cells that build new bone (*osteoblasts*) and cells that clear away old bone (*osteoclasts*). This setup may sound familiar if you've ever renovated a house. One crew comes in to knock down walls, and then (a month after the first crew trashed your house), another crew comes in to build a new room. Medical professionals refer to the bone-growing process as 'remodelling' because it serves the same purpose as remodelling a house. This lifelong, bone-remodelling process helps maintain healthy bone, fixing the wear and tear caused by everyday living.

At some point, a section of bone is selected as a remodelling site. (Scientists don't know much about how the site gets selected.) Osteoclasts remove bone by dissolving it with acid, which creates a cavity. This process of breaking down bone is referred to as bone *resorption*. What happens to the dissolved bone? The body is efficient at recycling and conserving resources – the calcium and other minerals from the resorbed bone pass into the bloodstream and are used in other parts of the body. In fact, whenever your body needs extra calcium, the osteoclasts get busy dissolving more bone – so best to keep your body well supplied with calcium so that your osteoclasts don't cannibalise your bones.

After the osteoclasts have done their thing, the osteoblasts get to work building new bone, and start spreading a gel-like substance in the cavity. Over the course of a month, this gel hardens into bone. The bone-remodelling project takes about two to three months. That's probably quicker than your last house renovation, but it's a slower healing process than those associated with other tissues such as muscle and skin.

Keeping Pace with Bone Reconstruction

Even after you reach your full height, your bones keep gaining and losing bone material. Your body's maintenance process, called *remodelling*, keeps your bones strong and healthy, day in and day out. Your hormones help regulate the maintenance process – and as your hormone levels change during menopause, the bone maintenance process messes up. (Check out the sidebar 'Remodelling your house of bones' for the ins and outs of bone remodelling.)

During your first 30 years on this planet, bone building exceeds bone destruction in the remodelling process, and your bones generally stay nice and healthy. After you reach the big 30 – or thereabouts, the teardown crew stays active, but the builders have a harder time keeping up.

The builders don't quite fill in all the cavities created by the demolition crew, and the maintenance process is now unbalanced. Like a washing machine with all the clothes clumped on one side, the cycle begins to break down. As the demolition crew destroys more bone than it repairs, your bones weaken and become less dense.

Making the calcium connection

Calcium is the central figure in the bone story. Your body needs calcium to build bones and to keep every cell in your body in shape. Calcium helps your muscles contract, your nerves to respond appropriately, and your blood to clot. Bones store the calcium your body uses until they release the calcium to a part of the body that requests it.

Table 4-1 lists calcium requirements by age. As your bones grow larger, your body needs more calcium. Your calcium requirements level off during your reproductive years as oestrogen helps your body absorb the calcium in your food. The figures given here are the UK reference nutrient intakes. Some nutritionists, however, believe that women need even more calcium than we list here, especially after the age of 50.

Table 4-1	Calcium Requirements by Age (UK Reference Nutrient Intakes)
Age (Years)	*Calcium Recommendation (in Milligrams/Day)*
1–3	500
4–8	800
9–10	1,300
11–18 (male)	1,000
11–18 (female)	800
19–50 plus	1,000
51 and older	1,200

When you eat a food or a food supplement rich in calcium, the calcium doesn't automatically go to your bones. First, calcium is digested and absorbed into your body to help your bones and other tissues that need it.

Attention pregnant and nursing mums

Your body demands even more calcium than normal during pregnancy and when you're breastfeeding. Although hormonal changes during pregnancy help your body absorb calcium more efficiently, if you're not getting enough calcium your body makes up for it by dissolving bone. If you have a multiple pregnancy or closely spaced pregnancies, ensure that you get enough calcium and vitamin D. Getting sufficient quantities of these nutrients usually requires taking food supplements in addition to pregnancy vitamins.

Breastfeeding, particularly for more than six months, also depletes your body of calcium. You have two concerns in this situation:

✔ You want to make sure that your milk contains enough calcium to nourish your baby properly.

✔ You want to make sure that the calcium supply comes from your diet, not your bones.

Fortunately, nature takes care of the first concern. Unfortunately, your bones may suffer as a result. If you don't have sufficient calcium for your baby, your body pulls calcium from your bones. Although they're controversial, some studies show that women can lose up to 5 per cent of their bone mass when they breastfeed. Again, calcium and vitamin D supplements in addition to pregnancy vitamins are critical.

You may think that keeping your bones building and rebuilding is simply a matter of getting enough calcium. But you also need a number of vitamins and hormones to help your body digest and absorb calcium properly (see 'Nutrition' later in this chapter for more on vitamins).

If the calcium in your blood drops below a certain level, your *parathyroid glands* get to work to help correct the situation. These glands monitor the amount of calcium in your blood; when the calcium level is low the parathyroid glands send parathyroid hormone into your bloodstream to deliver important messages to your kidneys and your osteoclasts.

✔ Your kidneys get the message: 'Save calcium! Don't put it in the urine!' In response, your helpful kidneys start activating the vitamin D they're storing so that you can better absorb the calcium you eat.

✔ Your *osteoclasts* (the bone destruction crew) get the message: 'Start mining calcium from the bones to beef up supplies in the bloodstream!'

Your body cannibalises its own bone to supply calcium to other cells if it doesn't get enough calcium or vitamin D. As a result, you suffer bone loss.

You have two ways to deal with this situation: Get more calcium in your diet or slow down the remodelling process so that the bone builders keep up with the bone destruction crew. You can get more calcium into your system through taking supplements and exercising. To slow down the destruction crew, you need medication (see 'Treating Osteoporosis' later in this chapter for more on drugs for osteoporosis).

Recognising the role of sex hormones

Your body needs vitamins to absorb calcium, but your sex hormones also play a big role in helping your body absorb the calcium that you eat and manage the remodelling process. Because your body produces less oestrogen after the menopause, your hormones are thrown out of balance. The imbalance affects your bones.

Oestrogen helps you absorb the calcium and magnesium you eat and deposits them properly into your skeleton to give you strong bones. Oestrogen also has a calming effect on bone destruction and lets the bone builders catch up with the bone destroyers. As your oestrogen supply dwindles during menopause, the bone destroyers get more active. What's more, you aren't able to digest as much of the calcium and magnesium that you get from your food as your oestrogen supply declines. If you continue eating like you have in the past, the same amount of calcium and magnesium won't go nearly as far in helping to build bone. That's why lots of women add calcium and magnesium supplements to their diet after menopause as a nutritional safety net, which is a good idea.

Other sex hormones that help in the bone building process include progesterone and testosterone, which your ovaries also produce.

- ✔ Testosterone is a better bone builder than progesterone. Testosterone not only triggers the osteoblasts to build bone, but also helps them to build stronger bones.
- ✔ Progesterone helps the bone builders repair bone, but only if oestrogen is present.

The slowdown of oestrogen and testosterone production during menopause is another reason why the bone builders have a hard time keeping up with the destruction crew after menopause.

So, sex hormones are an important player in the osteoporosis game because they regulate bone remodelling. If you let the bone destroyers get too rowdy and don't force the bone builders to keep up with them, bone deteriorates and becomes less dense.

Developments in oestrogen and osteoporosis

Cytokines may help us figure out how oestrogen slows down the bone destruction that leads to osteoporosis. *Cytokines* are substances inside the bone that regulate immune responses. Some of the latest research shows that cytokines may also regulate the osteoblasts and osteoclasts – the bone builders and destroyers.

So far, researchers know that levels of one of these cytokines, *interleukin-6*, rise after menopause. Scientists also know that the teardown crew (osteoclasts) becomes even more active after menopause if you don't take hormone replacement therapy (HRT). Putting two and two together, perhaps a rise in interleukin-6 causes the osteoclasts to more actively destroy bone. Oestrogen replacement reduces interleukin-6, and it also stops bone loss. Is this a coincidence? Scientists are trying to determine whether a connection exists and whether other interleukins are involved.

Understanding Osteoporosis

Osteoporosis is a disease, in which bones are weak and brittle. Bone deteriorates as you grow older, and if you live to a ripe old age you lose bone – all part of the natural ageing process. Not everyone with ageing bones develops osteoporosis, but this disease is a serious issue for many women – particularly during and after menopause.

The real danger of osteoporosis is that it sets the stage for literally breaking a leg (or a hip, or a wrist, or another bone). And as you age, breaking a bone becomes more than just an inconvenience – it can be deadly. A hip fracture carries the same mortality rate as breast cancer in older people, and half of all people with hip fractures are dependent upon caregivers for the rest of their lives.

Linking osteoporosis and women

We have good news and bad news about osteoporosis and women. The bad news is that about 2.1 million women in the UK have osteoporosis, of which around half a million are taking medication for the condition. The good news is that osteoporosis is preventable and treatable, even after menopause.

Women lose bone at wildly different rates, so the following generalisations reflect averages for the *perimenopausal* (premenopausal), menopausal, and postmenopausal years and don't necessarily apply to every woman:

- **Perimenopause:** Most women begin losing bone from their spine before or during perimenopause at a rate of 1 per cent per year.

- **Menopause:** After you are menopausal, the rate of bone loss increases to about 3 per cent per year if you don't receive hormone therapy.

- **Postmenopause:** At some time during the ten years following menopause, bone loss slows back down to a rate of about 1 per cent per year.

In the first five to seven years following menopause, you may lose as much as 20 per cent of the total bone you're expected to lose during your lifetime. By the time you're in your eighties, you may have lost as much as 47 per cent of your total bone density.

After reading all that, you may want more good news. Well, only 25–33 per cent of women develop osteoporosis. The idea of osteoporosis is like a weather forecast, though: You may have only a 33 per cent chance of rain, but if it rains on your picnic it's a mess.

Defining and diagnosing osteoporosis

Osteoporosis literally means porous bone – bone that is weak and brittle. Too little calcium in the bone is the cause of this disease. Both men and women can develop osteoporosis, but the disease is more common in women than men for a number of reasons:

- Women's bones are generally less dense than men's bones to start with.

- Testosterone stimulates bone growth and helps build stronger bones. Men have more testosterone – and therefore stronger bones – than women.

- Women tend to live longer than men.

In your grandmother's day, doctors diagnosed osteoporosis only if the patient actually broke a bone because of the disease. Waiting for a fracture before taking action is like buying a lottery ticket after the draw – it's a bit too late. Today, technology exists that can help identify osteoporosis before it results in painful, often debilitating fractures.

Diagnosing osteoporosis in terms of objective measurements of bone density is more practical than waiting for an injury. Bone-density measurements allow your medical team to treat your condition early so that you can prevent injury and promote healing. Modern, clued-up women are definitely into prevention.

How can you tell a healthy bone from a fragile bone? One way is to cut the bone in half and look at a cross-section (as we illustrate in Figure 4-1).

- ✔ A healthy bone looks like Swiss cheese – lots of cheese punctuated with small holes.

- ✔ A fragile bone looks like lace – lots of holes separated by thin, string-like threads of bone.

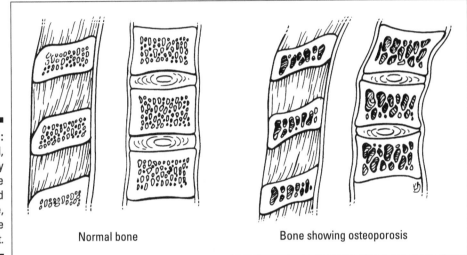

Figure 4-1: Normal, cheesy bone on the left and breakable, lacy bone on the right.

Normal bone   Bone showing osteoporosis

Medical types measure bone density (strength) to determine whether you have brittle bones. Nearly 30 years of research has proven that low bone density leads to fractures.

Osteoporosis today is defined in terms of how your bone density compares with the peak bone density of a healthy 35-year-old woman, which serves as the basis for the 'young adult' category in Table 4-2.

- ✔ If your bones are just slightly less dense than the bones of an average 35-year-old, the diagnosis is *osteopenia* – low bone density.

- ✔ If your bones are significantly less dense than the bones of an average 35-year-old, the diagnosis is *osteoporosis* – brittle bones. Table 4-2 shows typical criteria now used to diagnose osteoporosis.

Table 4-2	Criteria for Diagnosing Osteoporosis
Category	*Bone Density T-Score*
Normal	Less than 1.0 standard deviation below young adult
Osteopenia	1.0–2.5 standard deviations below young adult
Osteoporosis	2.5 or more standard deviations below young adult
Severe osteoporosis	2.5 or more standard deviations below young adult PLUS evidence of fractures

The threshold that separates osteopenia from full-blown osteoporosis comes from research that shows how much bone you can lose before significantly increasing your risk of fracture. If you have osteoporosis, you have low bone density, but you also have a higher risk of fracturing a bone.

Considering the causes of osteoporosis

Sixty years ago, doctors noticed that osteoporosis occurs primarily in menopausal women. They suspected that osteoporosis is related to sex hormones – specifically a deficiency of oestrogen. Hundreds of research grants later, we now know that oestrogen levels affect bone density.

Does menopause *cause* osteoporosis? The short answer is no. Osteoporosis is caused by calcium deficiency in the bones, and oestrogen plays a role in getting calcium to your bones and keeping bones healthy. (Check out 'Making the calcium connection' earlier in this chapter for more on calcium's role.)

Deficiencies of other vitamins, minerals, and hormones can influence the amount of calcium that your bone absorbs and therefore contribute to the development of osteoporosis. Lack of exercise can promote osteoporosis as well. Finally, lifestyle choices, such as the use of tobacco and alcohol, can also play a role in the onset of osteoporosis.

Avoiding the effects of osteoporosis

Osteoporosis weakens every bone in your body, leaving them prone to breaking. The bones most likely to break include those in your spine, hips, and wrists. Breaking your wrist may inconvenience you for a few weeks or months. Hip fractures are much more debilitating. And crushed vertebrae, so often associated with osteoporosis, can make you shorter and leave you with a stooped appearance.

✔ **Spinal fractures:** Fractures of the spine technically are not breaks but compressions. The weight of your body crushes, or compresses, the round body of the vertebra, giving these fractures their name, *compression fractures.* Compression fractures in your spine can leave you stooped with a hump in your upper back (a *dowager's hump*).

Between 5 and 15 per cent of 50-year-old women have compression fractures in their spine. By age 70, that number grows to between 40 and 55 per cent, depending on whose research you're looking at. Often, these crushed or wedged vertebrae cause little or no pain. You simply notice poor posture that you can't correct when standing up as straight as you can.

You may notice the first sign of crushed vertebrae during a routine medical examination. After you reach the age of 40 or 45, your doctor may start measuring your height. Women with crushed or wedged vertebrae are often shorter than they think they are. If you find yourself getting shorter, the measurement is not necessarily a mistake – it may be a sign of osteoporosis. Figure 4-2 shows the possible changes in your spine that accompany osteoporosis.

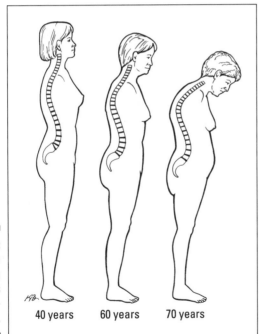

Figure 4-2: The shrinking effects of osteoporosis.

40 years   60 years   70 years

Although most women experience little or no pain when the vertebrae collapse, some women do. Over-the-counter painkillers such as ibuprofen and paracetamol can usually control the pain, which rarely lasts more than a few months. If pain is severe or prolonged, your doctor can prescribe stronger pain relievers.

✔ **Hip fractures:** This problem is generally the result of a fall that breaks the *femur,* the long bone of the thigh that connects your knee to your hip. The break often occurs at the head of the femur where it connects to the hip socket.

More than 90 per cent of hip fractures occur in people over the age of 70. So even though osteoporosis can begin during perimenopause, the effects are often corrected or held at bay through improved diet, exercise or medication, so you don't experience the debilitating aspects of the disease – the fractures. But don't underestimate the trauma of experiencing a broken hip at the age of 70. Only one-third of all women who have hip fractures regain the functionality they had before the fracture. Another third end up in nursing homes. And unfortunately, about 20 per cent die of complications within a year of the fracture. These life-threatening complications include blood clots and pneumonia, which can result from the immobility associated with hip fractures.

✔ **Wrist fractures:** Wrist fractures are common. When you fall, your first reaction is to catch yourself by sticking your hands out in front of you. You don't have to guess why wrist fractures are common in women with osteoporosis.

Preventing Osteoporosis by Managing Your Risk Factors

Your risk of developing osteoporosis is higher than your risk of getting breast, ovarian, or uterine cancer combined. After your 50th birthday, your risk of developing osteoporosis grows. One out of two white women over 50 will sustain a fracture due to osteoporosis in her lifetime. That's nearly twice as high as the fracture rate for black women. So, the next time you're out with your girl friends, look to one side: Depending on your ethnicity, it's likely that you or the woman next to you will break a bone in the future, thanks to osteoporosis.

Some women develop osteoporosis as they age, and others don't. Understanding why the disease happens can help you be one of the women who doesn't develop osteoporosis.

If you're a young woman you can start preventing osteoporosis today, as your bones keep gaining strength up until the age of around 30 years when you reach your peak bone density. If you're over 35, finding out how healthy your bones are right now is a good place to start. In both cases, prevention and treatment are easier if you understand how your bones stay healthy, how osteoporosis develops, and why your risk of developing brittle bones increases after menopause. (Check out 'Keeping Pace with Bone Reconstruction' earlier in this chapter for more on this.)

Risk factors for osteoporosis vary with age. From childhood through your twenties, you can lower your risk of osteoporosis if you get enough calcium, vitamins, and minerals, exercise regularly, and avoid unhealthy activities such as smoking and drinking too much alcohol. (See Chapters 19 and 22 for lots more on exercising.)

If you have children, whether they're toddlers or teenagers, encourage them to begin taking measures right away to prevent osteoporosis. The stronger your bones are early in life, the more you have to work with as you grow older. Having really dense bones when your bone density peaks (when you're about 30) gives you more bone to work with during and after menopause. Young people can develop strong bones if they eat properly and stay fit (see Chapters 18 and 19).

After your thirties are in your rear-view mirror and you begin to go through perimenopause and menopause, menopausal-related shifts in your sex hormones and other factors increase your risk of osteoporosis. (Check out 'Recognising the role of sex hormones' earlier in this chapter for more on the connection between osteoporosis and your hormones.) Risk factors boil down to three basic categories:

- ✔ Genetic factors and family background
- ✔ Personal health history
- ✔ Your lifestyle

We look at each of these topics in the following subsections.

Blaming your genes: Genetic factors and family background

Your genes establish a lot of the rules concerning how your body develops and how it ages. No surprise, then, that genetics plays a role in increasing or reducing your risk of osteoporosis.

White and Asian women have higher risks of osteoporosis than black women, particularly during perimenopause and the early years of menopause. Black women have a 6 per cent lifetime risk of osteoporosis, but white and Asian women have a lifetime risk of about 14 per cent. The lower incidence of osteoporosis in black women is probably due to the fact that black women have higher peak bone densities than white and Asian women. Even though everyone loses bone with age, black women have the advantage of inheriting stronger bones from the start.

Body build

Large-boned people generally build more bone than small-framed people, and they often start out with more bone mass when they hit their bone-building peak. As they age, large-boned people draw from a larger supply of calcium, so bone deterioration takes longer. But large-boned people aren't completely safe – some of them get osteoporosis too. Small-boned, or petite, women have lower peak bone densities, so they have less bone to lose.

Family history of osteoporosis

Scientists have found that daughters of women with osteoporosis tend to have lower peak bone density than normal for their age. Because of their genes, some women just don't make as much bone, even if they eat a proper diet and take exercise. Genes help determine our ability to make bone.

Reviewing your personal health history

A number of aspects of your personal history influence your risk of osteoporosis, including menstrual and menopause-related issues and the medications that you take.

Menstruation

Because oestrogen prevents bone loss, the more oestrogen you produce during your lifetime, the lower your risk of osteoporosis. Not surprisingly, many factors relating to your periods affect how much oestrogen you produce and, therefore, your risk for osteoporosis. Check out the following:

- ✔ **Age at your first period:** After you begin menstruating, your body produces more oestrogen. Most girls begin to menstruate between the ages of 11½ and 13. If you get your period early, you may produce more oestrogen in your lifetime than the average woman. With the additional oestrogen, your bones may have a higher peak bone density than the average woman. Of course, this statement assumes that you also eat a proper diet and take appropriate amounts of exercise. If you start out with higher bone density, you can lower your risk for osteoporosis.

✔ **Age at onset of menopause:** Most women go through menopause between the ages of 45 and 55. Women who go through menopause earlier, whether naturally or because of surgery, begin losing bone earlier than women who start the change later in life. You produce lower levels of oestrogen earlier, so your risk of osteoporosis goes up.

Your body produces much less oestrogen after menopause than it did during your reproductive years, and the more oestrogen you produce in your lifetime, the lower your risk of osteoporosis.

✔ **Ovary removal:** Women who have their ovaries removed (an *oophorectomy*) go through *surgical menopause*, which is exactly what it sounds like – immediate menopause caused by surgery. This sudden change jolts your system because you lose most of your hormones immediately and permanently. If you have your ovaries removed, you have twice as much bone loss and a higher risk of osteoporosis than women with their ovaries. If you have your ovaries removed before the age of 35, you may develop osteoporosis even if you take hormone replacement therapy (HRT).

✔ **Hysterectomy:** Women who have their uterus removed (*hysterectomy*) tend to go through menopause two years earlier than other women. The earlier onset probably results from cutting off part of the blood flow to the ovaries. The earlier onset of menopause increases your risk of osteoporosis a bit because you have fewer years of oestrogen production.

Eating disorders

Anorexia, bulimia, and over-exercising can lead to low oestrogen levels, which can cause you to skip periods and your body to begin losing more bone than it builds. Losing more bone than your body builds leads to osteoporosis.

Medications

Some medications affect peak bone density, raising your risk of osteoporosis. Ask your doctor and read the literature that accompanies the medications to determine whether you're at risk of bone loss from using a specific medication. The medications that can affect your bones include:

✔ Corticosteroids, used to treat chronic conditions such as asthma, rheumatoid arthritis, and psoriasis. These drugs increase bone loss as they inhibit calcium absorption. Women who take corticosteroid dosages greater than 5 milligrams daily, for more than two months, increase their risk of bone loss. Your doctor may also prescribe a bisphosphonate drug, such as alendronic acid, to slow down bone destruction and encourage bone building, if you need long-term steroids.

✔ Too high a dosage of thyroid-replacement medication or an overactive thyroid (as with Grave's disease). Excess thyroid hormone causes bone loss.

✔ Certain types of diuretics used to treat heart disease or high blood pressure, which cause the body to excrete more calcium. When used for prolonged periods of time, these drugs can raise your risk of bone loss.

Thiazide diuretics, on the other hand, actually reduce the amount of calcium excreted in the urine. They also seem to inhibit bone breakdown.

Surgery

Certain types of surgery can increase your risk of osteoporosis because they impact your body's ability to absorb or digest calcium or the vitamins and minerals needed to get calcium from your diet into the bone. These operations include:

✔ **Gastrectomy:** Removal of all or part of your stomach. This surgery decreases your ability to digest calcium and other nutrients needed to build bone.

✔ **Intestinal bypass:** Surgery to remove a portion of your intestine. This operation affects your ability to absorb calcium and other nutrients needed to build bone.

✔ **Thyroidectomy:** Surgery to remove part or all the thyroid gland. If your thyroid is removed, you must take thyroid-hormone medication. Too much thyroid-replacement medication triggers excessive bone loss and a decrease in bone strength.

Looking at your lifestyle

You can't do much about your age, even if you claim you're 39 years old for the rest of your life. But you can take steps to lower your risk of osteoporosis if you pick up a few new healthy habits and eliminate the unhealthy ones.

Age

From the time you're born until you're about 30, your main job is to build the strongest skeleton you can by eating a healthy diet, exercising regularly, and avoiding tobacco and alcohol. After you reach your thirties, your body loses bone faster than it can make it.

By the time you're 70, you've probably lost about as much bone as you're going to, but other aspects of ageing increase your risk of falling and breaking a bone. By age 70 or 80, your body has lost much of its flexibility, you may have less balance, your eyesight and depth perception are poor, and you may be taking medications that affect bone loss or physical conditioning.

Smoking

Smoking and using other tobacco products is unhealthy in every respect – not only because it decreases bone density. Tobacco use is especially unhealthy for children and adolescents. When children and adolescents smoke, they build less bone mass during a major developmental period in their lives. Because the use of tobacco decreases bone density, it's also not a healthy habit after menopause.

Alcohol

More than three units of alcohol a day is considered excessive as far as raising your risk of osteoporosis. Excessive alcohol consumption decreases bone density.

Exercise

Exercise is the kindest gift you can give your bones, apart from calcium. Exercise is critical for building strong bones. Exercise stresses your bones, which is a good thing as far as bone density is concerned. Stress forces the bone tissue to absorb calcium and therefore get stronger. Exercise also stimulates the muscles around the bone so that they get stronger and put even more pressure on your bones.

Interestingly, space research points to the importance of exercise in maintaining healthy bones. Scientists are concerned about the effects of prolonged weightlessness on astronauts' bones and encourage astronauts to exercise when they are in orbit.

Exercise during childhood and early adulthood is important in preventing osteoporosis because it helps your bones achieve their full potential strength. Later in life, exercise helps your bones to continue absorbing calcium so that they stay strong.

Lack of exercise not only decreases bone density but also makes you more susceptible to fractures. Women who exercise lower their risk of fracture as much as 30 per cent.

 Although physical activity helps protect your body against osteoporosis, too much strenuous activity can lead to low levels of oestrogen. Unless you're training for the Olympics, you probably aren't exercising too strenuously. Missing your monthly periods can be an important sign that you're over-exercising.

Nutrition

Calcium helps your body build bone. But calcium does much more than the TV advertisements proclaim. Calcium is also fundamental to regulating your sleep and moods and helping your muscles function properly.

Dairy products are the best source of calcium as far as food goes. A variety of vegetables also contain calcium, but vegetables contain less calcium per serving than dairy products. The fibre in certain vegetables makes it harder for your body to extract and use the calcium in them, but the form of calcium found in broccoli is more easily absorbed than that found in milk. For most women, consuming an additional pint of semi-skimmed or skimmed milk per day is a good compromise for gaining extra calcium (around 720 milligrams per pint) without consuming excessive amounts of fat.

Are soft drinks getting the best of you? Drinking carbonated soft drinks every day can zap the calcium out of your foods and supplements before it ever gets into your system. The phosphates in fizzy drinks bind with the calcium and magnesium, making them unusable. If you drink soft drinks regularly, increase your consumption of calcium. Doctors recommend that menopausal women get at least 700 milligrams of calcium every day after the age of 50 (check out Table 4-1 for more on daily calcium requirements). Drinking a pint of milk per day provides around 720 milligrams of calcium.

Many women find it easier to take calcium supplements than to get all the calcium they need from dairy products. With supplements, you know exactly how much calcium you're getting each day. Most nutritionists recommend taking calcium supplements that also contain vitamin D and magnesium, two other nutrients critical to healthy bone maintenance.

Check labels when choosing a calcium supplement, and avoid those made from oyster shell and dolomite, as these supplements may be contaminated with toxic heavy metals.

Adult women of all ages, but especially those who are postmenopausal should aim to get around 10 micrograms of vitamin D and 300 milligrams of magnesium every day to maintain healthy bones. Magnesium prevents bone loss as it plays an active role in bone growth. Magnesium also supports nerve cell communication (preventing wild mood swings), helps regulate blood pressure, and aids in muscle contraction. The last two functions help to prevent heart attacks. The heart is essentially one big muscle, so magnesium helps keep the contractions regular. Also, magnesium seems to prevent spasms of the blood vessels, particularly in the arteries around the heart.

Combined calcium and magnesium supplements help to prevent the constipation that some women experience when they take calcium supplements. Magnesium is a natural laxative and one of the main ingredients in milk of magnesia.

Vitamin K helps to prevent the body from cannibalising bone for calcium as it works to maintain proper levels of calcium in the blood. Vitamin K also produces a protein used to build bone called *osteocalcin.* You can get vitamin K by eating green leafy vegetables such as spinach and broccoli. You need between 0.5 and 1 microgram of vitamin K per kilogram of body weight – that's about 35– 70 micrograms of vitamin K a day if you weigh 70 kilograms (11 stone). 100 grams of broccoli contains about 117 micrograms of vitamin K, so you can easily get enough from your food.

Caffeine

Just two large cups of filter coffee (containing 300mg caffeine) causes you to lose an extra 15mg of calcium from your body. This may seem little, but it can contribute to as much as a 10% fall in bone mass over a ten year period. Women who drink four or more cups of filter coffee a day are three times more likely to have an osteoporotic hip fracture at some point in later life compared with non-coffee drinkers. Because coffee has more caffeine than tea and cola, curbing your coffee habit is one of the best ways to reduce your caffeine intake in your quest for healthier bones – try switching to decaffeinated beverages.

White tea contains around 15mg caffeine per average cup, compared to 20mg for green tea and 40mg for black tea. Instant coffee contains 60–70mg per instant cup; amounts are twice as high for strong drinks made with ground coffee.

Red Meat

Women who eat five servings or more of red meat each week increase their risk of fractures by as much as 20 per cent. Acids are sent into the bloodstream to help digest the protein and your body goes to the bones to supply calcium to neutralise the acids, which leads to bone loss. Vegetable proteins don't seem to cause the same responses as proteins from meats. So if you're going on a high-protein diet, try to get your proteins from fish and vegetables rather than from meat.

Finding Out whether You Have Osteoporosis

Most women who have osteoporosis don't feel anything unusual – it's a silent disease. Unfortunately, most women find out they have low bone density only after they've had a fracture. Other women first notice it in the mirror – their posture seems poor, even when they stand up as straight as they can. Other women have a chest X-ray for an unrelated reason and the doctor notices crushed or very thin vertebrae, indicating brittle bones.

One of the best ways to get a head start on avoiding this disease is to have a bone-density screening, a painless, non-invasive test. You simply lie down on a padded table, (usually you don't need to take your clothes off), and a machine passes over your body and records images. That's it!

To check out your bones, your doctor may recommend that you have a bone-density screening before the age of 40 and then routinely thereafter to measure your bone mineral density (often abbreviated to BMD) in two strategic locations – your spine and your hip.

Bone-density tests can help your doctor answer three important questions:

1. How much bone, if any, have you lost?
2. How quickly are you losing bone?
3. What's the best therapy to get your bones healthier and keep you from losing more bone?

The bone-density test produces a graphic image of your bones as well as statistics that compare your bones to healthy bones. You can find out how quickly you're losing bone by having these tests every two or three years. The results of your bone-density test will guide your doctor in choosing an appropriate therapy for bone loss if needed. These scans are available on the NHS if clinically indicated – for example if you have a strong family history of osteoporosis – and are available in private health-screening clinics too.

Doing the DEXA

To measure bone density, most physicians use a test called a *dual-energy X-ray absorptiometry*, or DEXA for short, which uses only a fraction of the radiation a chest X-ray uses.

Preparing an image of your hip takes only a few minutes and, for your spine, just a few minutes more. The technician can see the results immediately, although you often receive your report a few days later.

The report shows coloured images of your spine and hip reflecting different bone densities. The statistics that accompany the images compare your bone density with that of an average 35-year-old woman and with other women of your own age. (See the sidebar 'Reading a DEXA report' for more on understanding the test.)

Reading a DEXA report

The first thing you notice on the DEXA bone-density report is the colourful graphic image of your hip or spine. The technician generally tests both your spine and your hip, and the reports for each are nearly identical. We walk through the spine report here, but you can apply this information to your hip report as well. The *lumbar vertebrae* (lower back) are analysed for the spine test. The report you receive looks like an X-ray, but with colours corresponding to different bone densities. Typically, a legend shows the colour gradient going from low-density bone to high-density bone. This gradient allows you to see exactly where the low-density areas are sited.

Statistics that compare your *bone mineral density* (BMD) measurements with those of 35-year-olds are displayed adjacent to the image. You may wonder why your measurements are compared with a 35-year-old woman's measurements. And who is this 35-year-old you're compared with? Well, scientists have taken a large group of 35-year-old women, measured them, and used the average bone densities as a standard for comparison. When they compare your bone density to this 'standard', the difference is represented as a percentage. In other words, if your bones are half as dense as the average 35-year-old's, your statistics read 50 per cent; if your bones are the same, your statistics read 100 per cent.

Suppose your comparison shows that your bones are within 85 per cent of the 35-year-old. Is this fact terrible or terrific? To determine whether the percentage is statistically significant (something worth treating), the report includes a *T-score*.

T-scores show how many standard deviations your score is from 'normal'. In this case, *normal* is the score of a healthy 35-year-old woman of your ethnic background. Negative T-scores aren't so good.

A T-score of –1, isn't too bad (unless you have already experienced unexplained fractures). Your doctor will probably diagnose you with *osteopenia,* which means that you have low bone density (see Table 4-2 for the criteria used in diagnosing osteoporosis). If your T-score is –2.5 or lower, your doctor will probably diagnose you as having osteoporosis and recommend a course of treatment or some kind of dietary/fitness intervention.

When you begin losing bone (and everyone does), you need to figure out whether you're losing it slowly or quickly. Therefore, it's important to get a baseline test between the ages of 35 and 40 and to continue to monitor your bone density throughout your life. Most doctors recommend that you check your bone density about every two years. You can compare the most current results with the previous results to determine the rate of loss (or gain).

If you're at high risk for osteoporosis due to genetics or life events, we suggest you have your initial bone-density test during your early thirties and have subsequent tests every two years after that. Unfortunately, this level of screening is not yet available on the NHS and you are likely to have to pay for private screening.

Opting for another type of test

The DEXA bone-density measurement is probably the most commonly used procedure, but you or your doctor may opt for another procedure. Several devices work on the same principle as the DEXA bone scanner, including

- **Dual-photon absorptiometry (DPA):** Introduced in the early 1980s, DPA was one of the first devices to be able to measure bone density in the spine and hip – the best bones to use as predictors of total body bone density. Earlier devices couldn't measure density in bone covered by heavy muscle, so they were restricted to testing the wrist and heel.

  The DPA machine is a bit slower than today's DEXA – it takes about an hour to measure the hip and spine. Also, this machine isn't as precise as DEXA and can't measure small changes, so using it for comparisons is more difficult.

- **Quantitative computed tomography (QCT):** Also known as *CAT scanning* and *CT scanning*, QCTs can measure bone density anywhere in the body. The advantage of this procedure over the others is that it can accurately measure the centre of each vertebra in the spine. DEXA measurement can only measure a certain type of vertebrae because other bones are in the way.

  CAT scans typically aren't used to measure a patient's bone density on a yearly basis because it exposes the patient to more radiation than the other techniques – and they're pretty expensive.

- **Ultrasound:** This test is sometimes used to measure bone density in the heel and kneecap. These machines are portable, so theoretically they can screen more people using this quick, inexpensive bone-screening procedure. On the down side, this machine is limited to measuring bone density in *peripheral* sites – places other than the preferred spine and hip sites. If an ultrasound detects low bone density, you should have a follow-up DEXA test.

- **Urine tests:** As bone dissolves, some of the by-products show up in urine. When performed every few months, urine tests can tell whether bone loss is increasing or decreasing.

  Urine tests aren't an accurate diagnostic instrument for osteoporosis as you can have low bone density but lose bone slowly. Urine tests are generally used with patients on a treatment programme for osteoporosis to monitor progress.

X-rays are not used to test for bone density because changes in the 'whiteness' of the bone on the X-ray aren't detectable until you've lost 30 per cent of your normal bone mass. Clearly you want to take action before you lose 30 per cent of your bone mass.

Treating Osteoporosis

The first step in reducing bone loss is to eliminate unhealthy habits such as smoking and excessive alcohol use and to pick up healthy habits such as eating healthily and exercising regularly. Even the least invasive treatment programmes, such as calcium supplements and increased exercise, can slow bone loss and improve bone density.

More aggressive treatment programmes include bisphosphonate drugs and/or hormone therapies. These programmes can slow and even reverse bone loss. Many doctors recommend that women at high risk of osteoporosis begin hormone replacement therapy (HRT) during menopause. To prevent bone loss, you need oestrogen levels that are at least half of that occurring during a normal menstrual cycle. Some women with a significant amount of bone loss also add testosterone to their hormone regimen. Hormone replacement therapy (HRT) is ideally started early in menopause in addition to the other treatment programmes. For more information about osteoporosis, and its prevention and treatment, contact the National Ostopeoporosis Society (www.nos.org.uk; Helpline: 0845-4500230; e-mail: nurses@nos.org.uk).

Chapter 5

Taking Heart

. . . .

In This Chapter

▶ Getting the goods on 'good' and 'bad' cholesterol

▶ Uncovering oestrogen's connection to cardiovascular disease

▶ Laying out the risk factors for cardiovascular disease

. . . .

*W*hen it comes to matters of the heart, men and women are different (but you already knew that, didn't you?). Many men have their first heart attack between the ages of 45 and 55, but women usually don't have heart trouble until after they reach menopause (at an average age of 51). And, if a woman has a heart attack, she's more likely than a man to die from it. Why? One reason is that women have different symptoms than men. The crushing chest pains that warn men of heart attack aren't as common in women when they experience a heart attack. (The warning signs of heart attack for women are just a few of the many heart-healthy tips you can find in this chapter.)

In this chapter, we discuss heart attacks and many other types of cardiovascular disease. Your risk for cardiovascular disease increases after menopause because you lose the protective benefits of oestrogen. (We don't discuss *congenital* heart problems such as 'hole in the heart' in this chapter because these problems begin at birth rather than menopause.)

But the good news is, you can keep your heart healthy even after menopause. This chapter also discusses ways to keep your heart happy after the change – adopting a heart-healthy diet, getting a bit of exercise (well, ideally a lot) and eliminating bad habits.

Connecting Cardiovascular Disease and the Menopause

Oestrogen, the female hormone produced in the ovaries, is good for your heart. *Oestradiol,* the active form of oestrogen, is the most beneficial form of oestrogen, but (you guessed it) oestradiol is the type of oestrogen that decreases as you become menopausal. (Chapter 2 is full of information about what your hormones do.)

Basically, oestradiol is your secret weapon against all kinds of cardiovascular diseases. It's what every man wishes he has to avoid the early onset of heart problems.

Perhaps you've heard that before the age of 80, women are about half as likely as men their age to have heart disease. This statement leads many people to perceive heart disease as a largely male problem. It isn't. Men do tend to develop heart problems about 10 years earlier than women, so on average a woman has the heart of a man 10 years her junior. But just because men develop heart disease at an earlier age doesn't mean that heart disease isn't deadly for women. Just as many women as men die of heart disease each year.

Cardiovascular disease (disease of the heart and blood vessels) increases in women as oestradiol levels decrease. After menopause, your risk of cardiovascular disease shoots way up. Between 45 and 65 years of age, men experience three times more heart attacks than women. But after age 65, watch out – women have more heart attacks than men.

In order to give you the total picture, we include in this chapter information that you may not want to hear. Of all the ways a menopausal woman can pass into the hereafter, cardiovascular disease is the most likely culprit. In fact, after menopause, you're ten times more likely to die from cardiovascular disease than from breast cancer.

For some reason, word doesn't seem to have reached women and their doctors. Heart disease kills more women each year than breast, ovarian, uterine, and cervical cancers combined. To make things worse, the diagnosis of heart disease and heart attacks is often delayed in women as the symptoms aren't recognised and taken seriously.

The term *cardiovascular disease* (CVD) encompasses conditions that affect your heart and blood vessels, such as heart disease, heart attack, high blood pressure, coronary heart disease, and stroke. All these diseases restrict the flow of blood to the heart or brain.

Considering Your Cardiovascular System

Understanding how your heart and blood vessels work reveals the role that oestrogen plays in your cardiovascular system. In its simplest form, your cardiovascular system consists of your blood vessels and that big pumping muscle you know as your heart (see Figure 5-1). Oestrogen (in particular, the active form, oestradiol) does a lot to keep your blood vessels and heart healthy and free from disease. The following list of the ways that oestradiol protects you from getting an achy-breaky heart pulls together all the studies that are published on oestradiol and the cardiovascular system.

- ✔ Oestradiol dilates (widens) your blood vessels to lower your blood pressure.

- ✔ Oestradiol increases the good cholesterol and lowers the bad (more on these in the section 'Looking at lipids and considering cholesterol' later in this chapter).

- ✔ Oestradiol stops your platelets (sticky particles in your blood) clotting too quickly.

- ✔ Oestradiol acts like an antioxidant to stop fat deposits forming on the walls of your arteries.

- ✔ Oestradiol facilitates the release of a chemical that relaxes blood vessels, which helps reduce vessel spasms and increase blood flow.

Blood carries oxygen to the heart and picks up waste on the way back. Fatty blood can wreak havoc on your cardiovascular system.

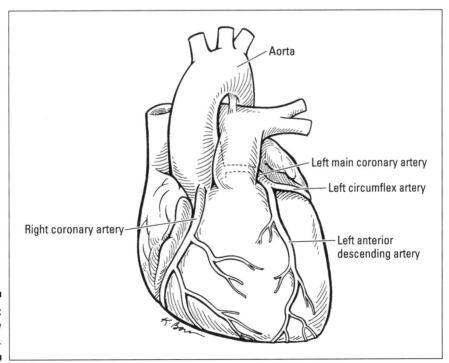

Figure 5-1:
The healthy heart.

Looking at lipids and considering cholesterol

From the time you reach puberty to the time you start menopause, you probably have a better cholesterol profile than a man of the same age. Women typically have higher levels of the good cholesterol (HDL) and lower levels of the bad cholesterol (LDL) than men during these years. But as you reach the menopause, your LDL levels rise and often exceed those of men your age.

Total cholesterol is not the total story for women. In men, higher levels of *total* cholesterol and heart disease go hand in hand. For women, the script is different. The *ratio* of LDL to HDL, as opposed to the sum of these two readings, is more important in predicting heart disease in women. The target ratio of LDL to HDL for women is 3.22 or less. The lower the ratio, the better. But a woman's HDL level is even more important than her LDL-to-HDL ratio. HDL levels in healthy women are over 1.79 mmol/L. (That unit of measure stands for *millimols per litre*, but you can just remember it as the unit medical types tack on to cholesterol test readings.)

The ball of wax that is cholesterol is broken down into various components:

- **Cholesterol:** At its basic level, *cholesterol* is fat – waxy, yellowish, oily fat. However, this fat (also known as a *lipid* in med- speak) is critical to keeping your well-oiled body running. Your body uses cholesterol to build and repair cells and to produce hormones, such as oestrogen and testosterone, vitamin D, bile (used to absorb fat), and myelin (which coats the nerves). If your blood contains too much cholesterol, the cholesterol gets deposited with other crud on the inside of your blood vessels. Cholesterol travels through your bloodstream on the back of proteins, so the particles are named *lipoproteins* – lipid plus protein equals lipoprotein. Lipoproteins with more protein than fat are called high-density lipids (HDL), and those with more fat than protein are called low-density lipids (LDL).

- **High-density lipids (HDLs):** These lipids are called the 'good cholesterol' because they help prevent the build-up of plaque. Because HDLs are mostly protein with just a little bit of fat, they have spare room to carry bad cholesterol back to the liver so that the body can flush it away.

- **Low-density lipids (LDLs):** Also known as the 'bad cholesterol', LDLs are mostly fat with only a small amount of protein. At normal levels, LDLs carry cholesterol from the liver to other parts of the body that need it for cell repair. When you have too much LDL cholesterol, it adheres to the walls of your arteries and attracts other substances. The combined glob is called *plaque*.

✔ **Triglycerides:** In addition to the fat known as cholesterol, your blood contains another type of fat – triglycerides – in small quantities. Triglycerides have little protein. They're almost pure fat, and the body uses them to store energy.

✔ **Total cholesterol:** This isn't another type of cholesterol. Rather, the term refers to a measure of the total amount of cholesterol (HDL plus LDL) in your blood.

To help separate the good cholesterol from the bad stuff in your mind, remember **Lousy DeaL**: Low-density lipids (LDLs) are the 'bad cholesterol' behind plaque formation.

You don't *need* to eat any cholesterol after your first year of life because your liver produces enough cholesterol on its own. Animal products such as meat, eggs, and dairy foods are especially high in cholesterol. Even though you don't need to eat these types of food to get enough cholesterol, most people enjoy meat, cheese, cake, and other stuff packed with cholesterol.

To find out the shape your blood is in, your doctor checks your cholesterol and triglyceride levels by taking a blood sample. The results, a *cholesterol profile* or a *lipoprotein analysis,* include your LDL, HDL, total cholesterol, and triglyceride levels. Using this information, your doctor can identify problems with your lipids and evaluate your risk of atherosclerosis (more generally known as hardening and furring up of the arteries).

The results from your cholesterol profile can help you determine whether your cholesterol and triglyceride levels are normal or off the charts. In Table 5-1, you can see about the ideal measurements for healthy cholesterol and triglyceride levels. If your results are outside these limits, your doctor may want to talk to you about improving your diet or taking medication.

Table 5-1	Ideal Cholesterol Levels (mmol/L)		
Total Cholesterol	*HDL*	*LDL*	*Triglycerides*
Less than 5	Greater than 1.2	Less than 3	Greater than 2.3

If you have diabetes, your doctor may set even stricter optimal blood fat levels. This is because people with diabetes have a higher risk of circulatory problems than normal, and research shows that they benefit from more tightly controlled blood fat levels.

Cholesterol: Following the process and looking at the factors

Most of us know that we are what we eat, but diet isn't the only thing controlling your blood cholesterol. Exercise, obesity, and age also influence your cholesterol levels and these factors are discussed in Chapters 18 and 19.

Your genes probably have the biggest influence on your cholesterol profile. Some women nibble on salads, avoid desserts, and rarely use butter but still have a cholesterol profile worse than that of someone who loves to eat cholesterol-intensive grilled cheese sandwiches and milk shakes when they're not snacking on a cream-of-something soup.

Regulating the role of oestrogen

Oestradiol (the active type of oestrogen) plays a major role in the way lipids are produced, managed, broken down, and eliminated from the body. Oestradiol also seems to help dilate blood vessels and keep them from having spasms. The lack of oestradiol is part of the reason why women are prone to cardiovascular problems after menopause.

Natural oestradiol is one thing, but hormone replacement therapy (HRT) is another when it comes to protecting your cardiovascular system. Take a look at Chapter 11 for more details on hormone replacement therapy (HRT), but here's the bottom line on hormones:

- **Combination hormone therapy:** Taking progesterone and oestrogen increases your HDL (good cholesterol) levels but also increases your LDL (bad cholesterol) levels and triglycerides.

- **Unopposed oestrogen therapy:** Only women without a uterus should take oestrogen alone (we explain why in a minute). *Oral oestrogen therapy* (without progesterone) increases HDL levels and decreases LDL levels. Unfortunately triglyceride levels tend to go up, which is not so good.

  The *oestradiol skin-patch* and oestradiol gel are examples of unopposed oestrogen therapy and, when used without progesterone, increase HDL and decrease LDL levels after about six months of use. The patch and gel also keep triglycerides in check.

When it comes to blood cholesterol, unopposed oestrogen therapy offers the best chance for improvement through hormone replacement therapy (HRT). Oestradiol patches when used alone provide the most beneficial results to date. But only women who have had their uterus removed should take oestrogen alone, as oestrogen without progesterone raises the risk of endometrial cancer in women who have a uterus.

Joining the dots between cholesterol and cardiovascular disease

If your artery walls are injured, perhaps as a result of smoking, cocaine use, diabetes, or other factors, your body may react too aggressively in repairing the walls. White blood cells come to the rescue and bring cholesterol with them to patch over the damaged area. After a while, other stuff adheres to the spot and the patch becomes harder, like a callus. The harder stuff is *plaque*. Reading the above, you can see how bad habits or disease can lead to hardening of the arteries – what your doctor calls *atherosclerosis*.

Sometimes people have far too much LDL cholesterol and not enough HDL to carry it out of their bloodstream. When this happens, LDL cholesterol gets deposited on the artery walls and rots. (Antioxidants can prevent the rotting, which is one reason why nutritionists suggest that you get plenty of antioxidants for a healthy heart.) Other substances then collect with the rotting cholesterol to form plaque. This is the process through which high cholesterol can lead to hardening of your arteries.

The latter process is like the build-up that causes your kitchen drains to clog. Rubbish goes down your sink every day, and every day a bit more gunk gets stuck on your pipes. Pretty soon the gunk slows down the water as it moves through the pipes.

With time, calcium begins to form on the plaque, hardening your arteries. Now your arteries are narrowed and hardened, and blood has a hard time flowing to the heart. Just as the water backs up in your sink pipes because of the clog, so the blood backs up in your arteries. Your heart then pumps harder to get the blood around your body. When your blood needs more pressure than normal, you have *hypertension* (high blood pressure).

Sometimes the plaque in your arteries breaks off and gets lodged in a blood vessel, as shown in Figure 5-2. Imagine pouring clog-busting chemicals down your drain, except instead of dissolving the clog the chemicals just loosen the gunk. Then the gunk gets stuck in the curve of the pipe. When a piece of plaque gets stuck in a blood vessel, the area of heart muscle that is fed via that vessel dies, and you have a heart attack.

Understanding Cardiovascular Diseases

A whole family of diseases affects your cardiovascular system, and a lot of inbreeding goes on in this family. For example, high cholesterol can lead to hardening of your arteries. Hardening of your arteries can lead to heart attack, stroke, and angina. Hypertension can lead to heart attack and stroke. In addition, your risk of all these conditions increases as your natural oestrogen levels decline after menopause.

In this section, we introduce you to the members of the cardiovascular-disease family. We also talk about preventing and treating unexpected visits from these conditions.

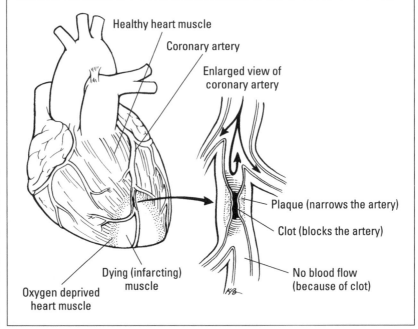

Figure 5-2:
The thing
to look at is
the clog on
the right.
Your heart
shouldn't
look like
this.

Labels in figure:
Healthy heart muscle
Coronary artery
Enlarged view of coronary artery
Plaque (narrows the artery)
Clot (blocks the artery)
No blood flow (because of clot)
Dying (infarcting) muscle
Oxygen deprived heart muscle

Containing coronary heart disease

Coronary heart disease (CHD) affects the blood vessels (the *coronary arteries*) that supply blood to your heart muscle. If these vessels are damaged, or if you have too much cholesterol in your blood, your coronary arteries become narrowed or blocked with plaque as cholesterol and calcium build up inside them. This process is called hardening of the arteries, or *atherosclerosis*. When your heart doesn't get enough oxygenated blood as a result of partially or totally blocked arteries, your heart muscle pays the price. The result is coronary heart disease. Coronary heart disease may cause angina (chest pain, which we talk about in the following section 'Avoiding angina') or a heart attack (check out the section 'Holding off heart attacks' later in this chapter). Around 1.15 million women in the UK have coronary heart disease, and over 124,000 British women have heart attacks each year.

Women often underestimate the severity of their chest pain or don't realise that their chest pain is related to heart problems. Therefore, they play down their symptoms when talking to their doctor. A couple of the reasons women give for not seeking help immediately are that they don't want to inconvenience anyone and that they think that heart disease is mainly a male issue.

Avoiding angina

To function properly, the heart muscle needs a constant supply of oxygen and nutrients delivered in the blood. If your veins or arteries are narrow due to a fatty build-up in the artery walls (atherosclerosis), you may experience the severe chest pain called *angina*. You feel pain because insufficient amounts of blood are getting through your veins into your heart muscle, and your heart is straining to pump enough blood to keep your body going strong.

Spasm in the blood vessels that take blood to the heart can also cause angina. Spasms can occur even if no blockages are present. Women are much more likely than men to suffer angina with no evidence of blockages.

Symptoms of angina sometimes begin during physical activity or emotional stress. Symptoms typically last about ten minutes and go away after several minutes of rest. But many women also experience chest pain as they rest. This pain is typically triggered by spasms or an *arrhythmia* (irregular heartbeat).

Angina is a very common early warning sign of coronary heart disease (CHD). Because CHD is so lethal in women, heart specialists typically schedule further tests right away for women with severe chest pains. (For more on coronary heart disease, check out the section 'Containing coronary heart disease' earlier in this chapter.)

Unfortunately, a survey studying how accident and emergency doctors treat patients with severe chest pain shows that men receive much more aggressive and quicker treatment than women. Also, men are twice as likely as women to have *coronary arteriography* (a special test that looks at the coronary arteries) and bypass surgery after complaining of chest pain. However, this is now starting to change in the UK as there is growing recognition among the medical profession that women are vulnerable to heart attacks, too.

Holding off heart attacks

Menopausal and postmenopausal women have an increased risk of heart attack (*myocardial infarction* in medicalese). Most women do not experience a heart attack until after the age of 60, but heart disease may start as early as the pre-teen years. Cholesterol accumulations are found in girls as young as ten years old. These accumulations in young children, called *fatty streaks,* sometimes turn into more significant build-up later in life.

Blocked arteries often cause a heart attack. Plaque breaks loose or a *blood clot* (a mass of solidified blood) blocks an artery, cutting off blood supply to part of the heart muscle. If the blockage remains in place for five to ten minutes or more, the piece of heart muscle fed through that artery begins to die.

Vessel spasm and arrhythmia are two additional causes of heart attacks, and evidence suggests that they're a more common trigger of heart attack in women than in men. *Spasm* constricts your coronary arteries so that blood can't get to the heart. Spasm can also cause plaque to break away from the vessel and get lodged in an artery, cutting off blood supply that way. *Arrhythmia,* or an irregular heartbeat, can mess up the pumping action of the heart and cut off blood supply as well.

Women often have different symptoms before a heart attack than do men. The symptoms of heart attack are easy to overlook because they're often subtle and typical of many other, less serious problems. Frequently, women say 'Oh yes, now that you mention it, I felt just like that yesterday' after a heart attack has already occurred.

Pay attention to warning signs. As a woman, you may not feel the typical crushing, squeezing, heaviness, or burning chest pain that many men feel before a heart attack. Instead, you may experience one or more of the following symptoms:

- ✔ Back pain
- ✔ Bloating
- ✔ Chest pain while resting
- ✔ Fatigue
- ✔ Heartburn or abdominal pain
- ✔ Jaw pain
- ✔ Joint pain
- ✔ Light-headedness/fainting
- ✔ Shortness of breath
- ✔ Sweating

An unfortunate by-product of a heart attack is a condition called *ventricular fibrillation*. This refers to an irregular heartbeat that occurs when the main pumping chambers of the heart, the *ventricles,* can't get coordinated properly; therefore, the blood can't get to the far reaches of the body so, for example, you may lose consciousness due to lack of oxygen and nutrients reaching the brain.

Heading off hypertension

High blood pressure is one of those health issues that's more likely to pop up as you get older. Until the age of 55, women usually have lower blood pressure than men. Between 55 and 65 years of age, women and men are about equal in the incidence of high blood pressure. After 65, more women than men have high blood pressure. So, just when you're dealing with all the symptoms connected with menopause, you may develop high blood pressure as well (your doctor may call it *hypertension*).

About half of all white women and three-quarters of black women over 50 have hypertension. For some reason, black women are more prone to hypertension than white women. The Asian population living in Britain is at higher risk of developing hypertension, too.

No one knows exactly why people develop high blood pressure. About 5 per cent of the time, high blood pressure is due to a condition such as diabetes or pregnancy, and it often can go away with treatment or resolution of the precipitating condition.

To visualise high blood pressure, think of blowing up a balloon. As you blow into the balloon, the air in your mouth is under a great deal of pressure because you're trying to pass it through the small opening in the balloon. Now, think of your heart as your cheeks and your arteries as the balloon opening – the smaller the balloon opening, the more pressure in your cheeks as you try to blow. So, if your blood vessels get smaller, perhaps due to cholesterol build-up, your heart has to pump harder to pass the blood through these narrower openings. The result: Your blood pressure rises.

High blood pressure can lead to heart attack, kidney damage, bleeding in the retina behind your eyes, and stroke. For these reasons, having your blood pressure checked routinely – ideally at an annual check, but at least every three years – is critical.

Many women develop high blood pressure because of obesity. Fortunately, these women can often reduce their blood pressure dramatically by switching to a heart-healthy diet (see Chapter 18), exercising regularly (see Chapter 19) and losing weight.

If you're not overweight, you may need to try other types of intervention. Some women are able to regulate their blood pressure if they reduce anxiety through meditation or other relaxation techniques. If these techniques don't work, medication is the answer to getting your blood pressure under control. You may have to work with your doctor to find just the right type of drug and dosage. One drug may work for some women but not for you. And, for some reason, drugs used to control blood pressure are more effective in men than women.

Staving off stroke

Stroke can occur for one of two reasons: A blood clot blocks the flow of blood to your brain or a blood vessel in your brain ruptures. In both cases, oxygen-rich blood can't get to the brain to nourish it. The problems a stroke causes depend upon the location and severity of the stroke, but speech problems, physical weakness, paralysis, and permanent brain damage are all possible complications. Many people having had strokes go through rehabilitation programmes that restore full or partial function to the affected areas of the body.

Symptoms associated with stroke include the following:

- Difficulty talking or understanding speech
- Dizziness
- Loss of vision, particularly in just one eye
- Unexplained numbness or weakness in the face, an arm, a leg, or one side of the body

A *transient ischaemic attack* (TIA) is like a mini-stroke. During a TIA, blood flow to the brain is interrupted (usually by a blood clot). The symptoms of a TIA usually last only 10 to 20 minutes and end when blood flow returns to normal. At worst, the symptoms of a TIA last 24 hours; symptoms of a stroke can last a lifetime. If you have any of the symptoms associated with stroke, contact your doctor immediately.

Pay attention to TIAs because they are often early warning signs of an impending stroke. Half of the people who have a TIA suffer a stroke within a year.

Recognising Risk Factors of Cardiovascular Disease in Women

Many of the risk factors for cardiovascular-disease-related complications are more risky for women (particularly menopausal women) than men, but many are risk factors for both men and women – including people who seem to be in good health.

- ✔ **Alcohol:** Women don't produce as much of the enzyme *alcohol dehydrogenase* used to break down alcohol as do men. So women tend to feel the buzz from alcohol earlier than men, and alcohol stays in their system longer. Three or four drinks a day cause a noticeable rise in your blood pressure. (We outline the dangers of high blood pressure in the section 'Heading off hypertension' earlier in this chapter.) In large doses, alcohol acts like a poison and kills heart tissue.

- ✔ **Cholesterol:** Low HDL levels and a high LDL-to-HDL ratio increase your risk for cardiovascular disease. After menopause, your HDL levels probably drop a little bit. A bigger change takes place in your LDL level. As you age, your LDL levels keep rising – especially between the ages of 40 and 60. So your HDL and LDL levels and your LDL-to-HDL ratio usually worsen as you get older.

- ✔ **Cocaine use:** Cocaine and crack are dangerous drugs. Whether snorted, smoked, or injected, cocaine seriously damages your arteries and heart. Here are a few conditions that cocaine and crack use can cause: Spasm in the coronary arteries, restricted oxygen flow to the heart, and arrhythmia. If you have had a previous coronary-related condition such as a *mitral valve prolapse* (heart murmur), cocaine can cause sudden death.

- ✔ **Diabetes:** High blood pressure, excessive weight, and inactivity can lead to adult-onset diabetes. Adult-onset diabetes is becoming more and more common worldwide and is a serious issue for menopausal women. Diabetes can cause a host of other problems, including increased risk of heart disease. Here's the scoop on women, diabetes, and cardiovascular disease:

  - Women over 45 are twice as likely as men of the same age to develop diabetes.

  - Women with diabetes are over five times more likely to have a coronary event, such as a heart attack or angina, than women without diabetes.

  - Women with diabetes are four times more likely to die from a heart attack than women without diabetes. In fact, 80 per cent of all people with diabetes die from a heart attack.

  Fortunately, adult-onset diabetes is often prevented or controlled through weight loss, exercise, and a healthy diet. (Head to Chapters 18, 19, and 22 for more on diet and exercise.) The main causes of adult-onset diabetes are:

- ✔ **Excessive weight:** If you weigh 10 per cent or more than your *target weight* (the ideal weight for people of your height and build), you're overweight. If you weigh 20 per cent or more, you're obese. Chapter 18 has a chart to help you determine where you are in relation to your target weight. For example, if your target weight is 46 kilograms (7 stone 3 pounds), you're overweight if you weigh 56 kilograms (8 stone 11 pounds) or more. Excessive weight increases your risk of high blood pressure, heart disease, stroke, and diabetes. Because excessive weight leads to many diseases and complications, losing this weight can lower your risk for many diseases and complications. Excessive weight is a huge and growing problem (no pun intended) – more than one-third of all women in the United Kingdom are overweight and almost a quarter are obese. This means that over half of all women weigh more than their ideal weight.

✔ **High blood pressure:** High blood pressure can lead to heart attacks and stroke as the increase in pressure stresses your blood vessels. Stress on your blood vessels constricts your arteries and may cause plaque to separate from the vessel wall and clog your arteries.

✔ **Inactivity:** For women, inactivity is the most common risk factor for cardiovascular disease. Most women have little time or chance to incorporate a workout into their busy schedules. Chauffeuring children, performing household chores, and working a 40- or 50-hour week may leave you with no time or desire to take a walk or attend an exercise class. But you need to make the time for physical activity: Physical activity is never a waste of time, because exercise lowers your risk of heart problems by as much as 50 per cent. Keep in mind that half of all women die from cardiovascular disease. Take a look at Chapters 19 and 22 for ideas on increasing your activity levels.

✔ **Personality:** Many people believe that too much stress results in high blood pressure and heart attacks. Research indicates that both control and stress are issues here. Women who feel in control of their lives are much less likely to have heart disease than women who feel they have little control. Cholesterol profiles are also much better in women who feel in control of their jobs, lives, and homes. When you feel out of control, you're more likely to feel cynical, hostile, or sorry for yourself – and researchers link these personality traits to a higher incidence of heart disease.

✔ **Smoking:** Cigarette smoking triples your risk of heart attack and angina. Even women who smoke fewer than five cigarettes a day double their risk of heart disease. When you inhale smoke, your heart beats faster, your blood vessels constrict, and your circulation slows down. The nicotine in cigarettes promotes blood clots (which can lodge in your arteries to cause heart attack and stroke). Smokers also have a greater risk of high blood pressure and emphysema, an unpleasant lung disease.

Being Smart about Your Heart

Eating a healthy diet, watching your weight, exercising routinely, avoiding unhealthy habits, and having annual medical examinations are the best ways to prevent cardiovascular problems.

Weighing an ounce of prevention

Keeping your blood clean and lean really helps prevent hardening of your arteries, which is the source of many serious problems. Controlling your cholesterol boils down to eliminating unhealthy habits (smoking, drinking too much alcohol, using recreational drugs, and so on), sticking to a healthy diet (check out Chapter 18 for the low-down on healthy eating), and exercising five days a week for half an hour (turn to Chapters 19 and 22 for more information on exercise).

If you're not able to control your cholesterol through lifestyle changes, you and your doctor can consider alternatives. A variety of medications are available that can lower your cholesterol.

Many people develop hypertension even though their cholesterol levels are terrific. A good doctor checks your blood pressure almost as soon as you step in the door. So keep those doctor appointments and, if your blood pressure is high, seek help. Work with your doctor to find the right drug for you – but remember that you need to take the medication every day for it to work.

Routine check-ups at least once a year with your general practitioner should prevent cardiovascular problems from sneaking up on you.

Treating what ails you

If you maintain regular appointments and seek help when you feel any weird happenings in your heart, such as palpitations or pain, you are following the safest route for long-term health. Of course, you also need to follow the advice your doctor gives you. If you have high blood pressure, take your medication as prescribed. Even though you usually have no symptoms with hypertension, not taking your medication can cause trouble. The same goes for high cholesterol levels: Many people have no symptoms when their cholesterol is high, but without treatment faulty cholesterol levels cause a world of problems.

A huge variety of medications are available to treat the conditions that we describe in this chapter. You and your doctor may need to experiment a bit to find the medicines that work for you, but the effort is worthwhile as the reward is a better quality – and quantity – of life.

Chapter 6

Making Sense of Vaginal and Urinary Changes

*1*f you have difficulty talking to your mum about menopause, imagine talking to her about the vaginal and urinary problems associated with the change. Not going to happen? You're not alone. Many women live with pain and discomfort because they're too embarrassed to discuss these problems with anyone – including family members, friends, and doctors.

You may notice that your vagina isn't performing its lubricating duties like it used to when you think about sex. Or perhaps sex is a bit uncomfortable. Your vagina feels dry, and you may experience itching around your vulva or in your vagina, a watery vaginal discharge, or a burning sensation when you urinate. The medical term for this condition is *atrophic vaginitis* or *vaginal atrophy*.

Vaginal and urinary issues are not unique to menopausal women – some women experience vaginal dryness during sex long before they're menopausal (especially if they're on the pill), while other women zoom past the menopause for several years without encountering vaginal dryness. Some women experience vaginal irritation only temporarily; others find it gets worse with age. Vaginal issues are, quite simply, a highly individual thing.

If you live long enough, without hormone therapy or some type of treatment your vaginal lining becomes thin and drier, but you may never experience any of the symptoms, pain, or discomfort. You may never even know what's happening. Some women notice dryness during sex or itching that lasts a few months while their body adjusts to the lower oestrogen levels. Other women experience discomfort during sex at first and then more intense symptoms as time goes on. If you do experience discomfort, don't simply put up with it – many effective treatments are available.

Your urinary tract and your female organs are located next to each other, and both systems rely on oestrogen to function properly. These two facts explain why problems can arise in both systems during the change and why changes in your vagina may affect your urinary tract.

Doc, Can We Talk?

Before you do anything about urinary-tract or vaginal problems, you need a doctor to diagnose your condition. Many problems exhibit symptoms that have nothing to do with menopause, so seeing a medical expert is a good idea.

You may think that telling your doctor about painful sex or problems with your plumbing is embarrassing, but get over it. Your doctor's heard it all before. In fact, medical books warn doctors that patients under-report these problems due to embarrassment. Doctors are supposed to raise the issue of intimate problems themselves, but they often don't – not because they're too embarrassed, but due to lack of time or forgetfulness. So bring 'em up yourself.

Here are a few tips for talking about your symptoms:

✔ **Keep a diary:** Plan ahead for your visit to the doctor. If you experience vaginal or urinary tract pain, keep track of when it hurts, where it hurts, the presence or absence of discharge, the colour of the discharge, and any other details. If you experience urinary leakage, write down what time you tinkled, how much urine was involved (use any measure you're comfortable with – cups, ounces, teaspoons, whatever – and let the doctor do the maths). What triggered the accident? Did you lose it when laughing, exercising, sneezing, or watching TV? Also note any type of discomfort and the level of pain.

✔ **Be specific:** When discussing things with your doctor, don't just say that you're uncomfortable 'down there' and then lift your eyebrows to make your point. Tell the doctor what symptoms you're experiencing.

✔ **Be persistent:** If the doctor's response isn't helpful – 'That's normal for women your age' – press the issue to get the advice and help that you need to deal with the problem. Just because 'it's normal' doesn't mean there's no treatment.

Vaginal Atrophy and Other Issues

Many women fear the natural result of menopause is for their vagina to dry out, shrivel up, and become a sexual wasteland. This doesn't have to happen. In fact, *less than half* of all postmenopausal women complain of vaginal dryness or other symptoms of vaginal atrophy.

The term *atrophy* may make you think of stagnant, dead things such as those plump little worms that get stranded on a pavement after a rainstorm and end up dried out and dead. The dictionary defines *atrophy* as 'wasting away' and 'failure to grow because of lack of nutrition'. But vaginal dryness isn't an insurmountable problem, and we're here to tell you how to deal with it.

Vaginal changes accompanying the menopause don't have to make you uncomfortable or make sex unappealing. You can find many ways to keep your vagina pliable and moist so that sex continues as a normal and enjoyable part of your life. All menopausal women experience vaginal changes, but you can reduce the unwanted side effects.

What it is and what it isn't

Because oestrogen keeps your vagina moist and elastic, loss of oestrogen can make your vagina drier, thinner, and less elastic. The downturn in oestrogen production that comes with menopause can also cause your vagina to shrink slightly in width and length.

An atrophic vagina loses some of its plumpness and firmness because the lining is thinner and doesn't have the furrows and folds typical of a fertile vagina. (Yes, this is one case in which wrinkles are a sign of youth.) The vagina appears red instead of pink. Also, with less mucus, the vagina is less acidic, so it's easier for bacteria to grow, which causes the watery discharge that some women experience.

Talk to your doctor about vaginal changes if you experience discomfort. Dryness and other vaginal-atrophy-related symptoms may prompt you to avoid sex just when you have more time for it. Don't avoid bringing it up – your doctor knows of plenty of easy ways to fix this one.

What lower oestrogen means for your vagina

Oestrogen is the secret behind keeping your female organs working like a well-oiled machine. Oestrogen bathes your vagina and your urinary tract, keeping the tissues lubricated and flexible. As your oestrogen levels start to fall during menopause, the following things happen:

✔ Your vagina becomes more susceptible to tears and damage from friction.

Sexually transmitted infections have an easier time invading your body through tears than through an intact lining. So, step up your protection after menopause if you're with new or multiple partners. Also, because tearing your vagina is easier after menopause, watch the rough stuff.

✔ As vaginal tissues lose their elasticity, your vagina becomes less pliant and sometimes smaller. Sex is sometimes less enjoyable if you don't intervene with some type of therapy such as a simple lubricant or hormone replacement therapy (see the section 'What to do about it' later in this chapter).

✔ Your vagina may not produce the lubricating fluids during sexual arousal it did before menopause, so if intercourse is painful, use a lubricant.

✔ Mucus maintains your vaginal acidity, which destroys much of the bacteria introduced into the area through sex and wiping after you go to the toilet. When your production of vaginal mucus tails off, infections find it easier to grow, and you are more susceptible to an overgrowth of vaginal bacteria, leading to *bacterial vaginosis* (inflammation of the vagina caused by an abnormal bacterial balance).

What to do about it

For some women, the easiest way to prevent or slow down the progress of vaginal atrophy is regular sexual activity. Sexual activity increases blood circulation and lubrication and promotes vaginal elasticity. If you don't have a sexual partner, masturbation provides the same benefits.

If dryness inhibits your sexual desire, try one of the many lubricants available over the counter. Some of the lubricants are for use during sexual activity; others act like a moisturiser and cause your vagina to absorb water. Some women also find that vitamin E relieves dryness. Break open a capsule and apply the oil directly to your vagina. If the vitamin E seems to make you sore, stop using vitamin E, as you may have a sensitivity to vitamin E products.

If you're using latex condoms or a diaphragm, only use water-soluble lubricants as those that are oil-based quickly weaken latex rubber. Check whether oestrogen creams and gels are suitable for use with condoms, too.

Applying oestrogen cream to the vagina also provides relief from the pain and itching associated with vaginal dryness. Vaginal oestrogen creams are more effective than oral hormone treatments for relieving discomfort due to dryness. Although most of the oestrogen stays in your vagina, some is absorbed into your bloodstream. However, doctors usually prescribe such a low dosage for this problem that using a vaginal oestrogen cream shouldn't substantially increase your risk of endometrial cancer or breast cancer like oral oestrogen does. In fact, vaginal creams are often prescribed for women who don't want to take hormones orally because they're at higher risk of endometrial or breast cancer.

As with hormone replacement therapy (HRT) and oestrogen pills, you need a prescription from your doctor for these creams.

You can use a lubricant during sex in addition to the oestrogen cream to keep things slippery.

Before we change subjects, here's one last tip: Drinking plenty of water keeps your entire body hydrated, including your vagina. Think of yourself as an athlete in training and try to follow an athlete's regimen: Drink more water. Drink less alcohol and coffee.

Hold It! We Need to Talk about Urinary Problems

A healthy urinary tract depends on healthy tissue and toned muscle around your plumbing. About 40 per cent of women between the ages of 45 and 64 have urinary-tract problems, which mainly take the form of *incontinence* (inability to hold back urine). You may never have a urinary-tract problem, but if you do you'll know the basics after reading this chapter.

Urinary-tract problems are not hidden away in the closet. Many products are available to help control or eliminate urinary disorders so you can enjoy all the activities in which you've always participated. Ask your doctor about appropriate courses of treatment.

Your *urinary tract* moves liquid waste from your kidneys, through your bladder, and out of your body. The tract consists of your kidneys, bladder, two *ureters* (the ducts that carry urine from the kidneys to the bladder), and urethra.

Urinary tract conditions are more common in women after menopause. The end of the *urethra* (the little tube from which your urine flows) is more dependent on oestrogen than any other part of your urinary tract. After menopause, when oestrogen is low for a period of time, your urethra can become inflexible. Simultaneously, the collagen and connective tissue (the fleshy stuff) around your urethra that supports your plumbing gets thinner. So two problems can occur:

✔ With less flexibility and thinner tissue in and around your urethra, you're more likely to get some microscopic tearing that makes it easier for bacteria to enter the urethra. Therefore, urinary tract infections (UTIs) develop more easily.

✔ The urethra has a harder time sealing itself using pressure, so you may leak or dribble urine when you least expect it and have instances of incontinence.

Nearly one in six women over the age of 45 develops one of these urinary-tract problems, so don't feel embarrassed when you talk to your doctor. These problems are quite common and highly treatable. Infections usually get worse with time, so go to the doctor right away if you think you've got plumbing problems.

Take a look at the section 'Doc, Can We Talk?' earlier in this chapter for tips on recording your symptoms in preparation for your visit to the doctor. Your general practitioner may refer you to a specialist gynaecologist or urologist, but your general practitioner can handle most urinary issues. In the following sections we tell you a bit about the common urinary conditions and what your doctor may do about them.

Tracking urinary tract infections

A whole slew of urinary tract infections (UTIs) are out there, but one thing they all have in common is that they're mainly caused by bacteria entering your plumbing through your urethra.

The most common UTI, *cystitis,* affects your bladder. Women are more prone to bladder infections than men because women wipe after using the toilet. Wiping can sweep germs from your faeces (bowel movements) into your urethra. These bacteria (especially *Escherichia coli,* more commonly called *E. coli*) can travel all the way to your bladder, or further into your kidneys, and cause an infection. Wiping from front to back reduces your chances of developing a UTI.

Frequent or vigorous sex can harm the delicate tissue of the vulva and outer urethra, which in turn allows bacteria into the body causing urinary tract infections. Sex can also push bacteria up into the urethra. Peeing immediately after sex helps you avoid UTIs.

Getting a diagnosis

A urinary tract infection usually starts with a burning sensation or pain when urinating, together with urgency, frequency, or both. *Urgency* refers to feeling like your bladder is so full it's about to burst and you can't make it to the toilet. *Frequency* is the feeling that you have to go to the toilet constantly.

If you have a UTI, you may find yourself rushing to the toilet, releasing just a trickle of urine, and then, a short time later, feeling as if you have to go again. This pattern is especially irritating at night. Repeatedly waking up to shuffle to the bathroom can leave you exhausted.

You may also notice that your urine is cloudy, has blood in it, or smells different from usual. If the infection is in your kidneys, you may have a fever, chills, back pain, nausea, or vomiting.

Urgency, frequency, and pain related to peeing are also symptoms of other conditions. If you experience any or all these symptoms, make an appointment with your doctor. Your doctor may ask you to do the tinkle-in-a-cup routine so that the professionals can examine your urine to determine whether you have a UTI or another condition. The tests your doctor may run include the following:

- ✔ **Dip-stick analysis**: Your doctor dips a stick into your urine and assesses the colour changes on several small chemical pads to look for hidden red blood cells, white blood cells, proteins, and bacteria.

- ✔ **Microscopy and culture:** Your doctor sends your urine sample to a laboratory for examination under a microscope, looking for white blood cells (which indicate an infection) and bacteria. The sample is also cultured to find out exactly what type of bacteria are present and which antibiotic is most likely to kill them.

Trying treatments

Treatment of a UTI usually includes a short course of antibiotics and directions to drink plenty of fluids.

Drinking several glasses of unsweetened cranberry juice every day helps your recovery from a bladder infection. Cranberry juice makes your urine more acidic, thereby making bacterial growth more difficult. Cranberry juice also contains substances called anti-adhesins, which stop bacteria sticking to the wall of your urinary tract.

Don't use cranberry juice as an alternative to visiting your doctor if you think you may have a urinary tract infection. Dangerous conditions such as septicemia (blood poisoning) can develop if a urinary tract infection is left untreated.

Introducing interstitial cystitis

Interstitial cystitis (IC) is often overlooked or misdiagnosed as a urinary tract infection because the symptoms are so similar.

IC affects as many as 2 per cent of women. Although IC occurs mostly in women after the menopause, some women develop IC in their twenties or thirties. IC affects some men too.

No one knows exactly what causes IC, but research suggests that frequent bladder infections make the bladder attack itself, leading to IC. Alternatively, an as yet unrecognised bacterium may attack the bladder lining. Some medical professionals also suggest that there's a link between reducing levels of oestrogen and IC.

Tissues in your bladder and throughout your urinary tract rely on oestrogen. Your nerve endings also need oestrogen. When oestrogen bathes your nerve endings during your reproductive years, you don't notice any sensation in your bladder until it's quite full, because oestrogen keeps your sensory threshold high. But, when your oestrogen levels reduce during perimenopause and menopause, your pain threshold is lower and you are more sensitive in your bladder area. Here are more clues that suggest a possible role for hormones in connection with IC:

- ✔ The average age of a person with IC is 44 years.
- ✔ Premenopausal women with IC seem to have recurrences during the part of the menstrual cycle when oestrogen levels are falling.

Getting a diagnosis

Interstitial cystitis is a specific type of bladder inflammation. Bacterial infections cause most bladder inflammations (known generically as *cystitis*), but if you have IC, your doctor won't find any bacteria when analysing your urine sample. So, it's not surprising to find out that antibiotics don't help with this condition. A lot of the symptoms of IC are similar to those of a bacterial bladder infection, including frequent urination (especially at night), sudden urges to urinate, and pain that becomes worse as your bladder fills. Sometimes the pain, which can get intense during urination, subsides after urination. The symptoms may go away from time to time and it's all a bit of a mystery.

Sometimes the pain is pretty generalised and occupies your entire pelvic area. You may feel pressure, tenderness, or pain in your bladder and the area around your bladder. If you're still menstruating, the pain may get worse just before your periods. You may also have pain during sex.

Diagnosing IC isn't easy. In their search for a cause of your symptoms, doctors initially go through a process of elimination, testing for UTIs and other conditions. After they eliminate these other possible causes, your doctor may take a peak at your bladder by inserting a scope through your urethra into your bladder (*cystoscopy*) to look for scarring or microscopic tears on the walls inside your bladder.

Trying treatments

The treatment options range from the least invasive – modifying your diet – to the most invasive – bladder surgery to repair the walls or, in desperation, removal of the entire bladder.

Some women find that eliminating certain items from their diet and lifestyle helps to relieve bladder irritation. These include alcohol, coffee, tobacco, sharp cheeses, artificial sweeteners, preservatives, and acidic foods. Dyes used in food and medicines can also irritate the bladder or cause bladder spasms.

Between modifying your diet and having surgery, you may find success by using mild analgesics to help manage the pain such as paracetamol.

Antibiotics are ineffective in treating IC. Women misdiagnosed with a urinary tract infection find that the antibiotics prescribed for that condition do little to help relieve the symptoms of IC.

Encountering incontinence

Three-year-olds have a hard time 'holding it' when they don't recognise the signal telling them that they have to tinkle, until it's too late. Later in life (after babies, surgery, and menopause) some women have trouble 'holding it' again, but for different reasons this time. Sometimes, your body just doesn't follow the orders your brain calls out.

When you can't hold back urine, or urine leaks out when you don't want it to, you have urinary *incontinence*. Lower levels of oestrogen contribute to lower muscle tone in your urethra, so that you lose bladder control. Weakening of muscles after bearing children or having surgery can make the problem even worse.

The urethra (the tube through which urine flows from the bladder out of your body) is controlled with a valve that keeps more pressure around the urethral tube than in the bladder, keeping the urethra closed. Oestrogen helps increase muscle tone, which leads to increased pressure, and prevents leakage. With lower oestrogen levels, the muscle fibres lose their flexibility and the urethra has a hard time making a tight seal where it connects to the bladder.

Getting a diagnosis

Incontinence comes in a couple of varieties:

- **Stress incontinence:** Urine may leak out when you laugh or sneeze or cough. Many women whose pelvic muscle tone is poor due to bearing children or having surgery suffer stress incontinence.

  The *stress* in *stress incontinence* has nothing to do with psychological pain. Rather, the *stress* refers to stress in your abdomen. When you cough or laugh, the pressure in your abdomen increases, which puts pressure on your bladder, so the bladder pressure is greater than the urethral pressure. Then laughing, coughing, and other activities such as running and trampolining set off a chain reaction that ends in leakage.

  About a third of women with stress incontinence are premenopausal. Unfortunately, after menopause, stress incontinence can get worse.

- **Urge incontinence:** This is less common than stress incontinence. With urge incontinence, you feel a tremendous urge to urinate, but before you get to the bathroom you begin leaking. You get 'caught short' because you just can't make it to the bathroom fast enough.

  Spasms in your bladder cause this type of incontinence. Urge incontinence is sometimes linked with more serious medical problems such as a herniated disc in your back, *fibroids* (little, non-cancerous wads of tissue), nerve damage, or even bladder cancer. Contact your doctor right away if you have urge incontinence so he or she can check out the condition.

Trying treatments

See your doctor if you experience any type of incontinence, as the incontinence is often a symptom of another medical condition. Treating the symptom is not always the best way to treat the whole disease.

Incontinence due to weakened muscles in the pelvic floor is treated with pelvic floor exercises – also known as *Kegel exercises* – which strengthen the muscles around your urethra. If you went to childbirth classes, you may have heard of these exercises. But Kegels are just as useful in menopause as they are after childbirth.

Strengthening the muscles supporting the urethra keeps you from leaking urine when you laugh, cough, and exercise. Kegel exercises also improve the muscle tone in your *pubococcygeus* (PC) muscle – the muscle you use to stop urine from flowing.

The biggest problem with Kegels is that most women aren't taught the right way to do them, so they don't get the full benefit. The sidebar 'Kegel in three easy steps' starts off your Kegel programme on the right foot.

Kegels can improve your muscle tone, but they don't strengthen thinned tissue. If thinning tissue is the cause of incontinence, surgery is often the appropriate treatment.

Other methods that you can use to handle incontinence due to weakened muscles include the following:

- ✔ **Pads:** These pads are similar to the pads you wear during your menstrual period. The pad absorbs leaked urine, and you change a used pad when you go to the toilet. These are available from pharmacies.

- ✔ **Silicone caps:** These caps, inserted into the urethra, seem to reduce leakage by about 50 per cent. Your doctor can advise whether this may help you.

- ✔ **Teflon, collagen, and dextranomer/hyaluronic acid injections:** Some urologists offer these injections to strengthen the tissues around the urethra or bladder neck by making them thicker. You normally need multiple injections.

- ✔ **Vaginal cones:** This approach uses little weights to strengthen your muscles related to controlling urine flow. You insert a tampon-like cone into your vagina and hold it there. The goal is to gradually increase the weight and the amount of time you hold the cone in place.

- ✔ **Vaginal exercisers:** You insert a progressive resistance device into the vagina and squeeze against it to help strengthen your vaginal muscles.

Talk to your doctor about these solutions and others, such as electrical stimulation and vaginal urethral rings. Medications are available that inhibit bladder contractions, help stabilise the bladder lining, or relax smooth muscle in both your urethra and bladder – all can help curb symptoms of incontinence. These medications include propantheline, flavoxate, oxybutynin, and imipramine – all control bladder spasms. These treatments are only available on prescription and your doctor can advise which, if any, is likely to suit you.

Kegel in easy steps

Every time you go to the bathroom, end the outing with a series of Kegel exercises. Although medical professionals usually say you only need do these exercises three times each day, you won't have to tax your memory if you just do them every time you urinate. If you follow this advice, you ensure that you're exercising routinely and frequently – two requirements for successfully strengthening the pubococcygeus (PC) muscle, which helps you stop urine from flowing. Here are the three steps to a stronger PC:

1. As you urinate, squeeze the muscle you use to stop the flow of urine. Now that you've found your PC muscle, you're ready for the workout. (Only do this initially to identify the PC muscle. Don't do it once you know which it is as doctors have some concern that starting and stopping the flow of urine midstream may help bacteria enter the urethra.)

2. Squeeze the PC muscle for three seconds (one one-thousand, two one-thousand, three one-thousand) and then relax for five seconds. Try to squeeze only your PC muscle, keeping your thigh, abdomen, and buttocks muscles relaxed. Squeezing the other muscles actually works against the exercise because it creates pressure above the urethra, which makes it difficult to squeeze the PC muscle. Do this exercise five times at the end of every visit to the bathroom.

3. Work up to holding each squeeze for 10 seconds and relaxing for 5 seconds in between squeezes. Continue doing five of these each time you go to the bathroom.

4. Contract the muscle at least eight times and do this at least three times a day. Carry on for at least three months to start with, and continue them if they help.

5. After six to eight weeks, many women notice an improvement in their ability to control the flow of urine.

If your sleep is interrupted by incontinence, and you restrict the amount of fluids you drink after dinner, make sure that you drink enough fluid during the day to make up for the curfew.

Chapter 7

Surveying Surfaces and Sinuses: Your Skin, Hair, and Nasal Cavities

*N*o, you're not going crazy or losing your mind if you think your skin is getting drier over the years. Face it – dry skin happens. And that dry skin is possibly related to menopause. Depending on which scientists you believe, the sags and wrinkles in your face are or are not due to lower levels of oestrogen. In this chapter we give you both sides of the story.

How are your sinuses doing? Do you seem to have a runny nose more often since turning 40? Guess what? This annoyance is tied to menopause as well. And, if as a child, you watched an aunt or grandma in total amazement, wondering how that one hair on her chin got so long – the menopause can explain that, too. Read on to find out why the hair on your head seems to migrate to your chin after the change.

No one is going to win a Nobel Prize for discovering a pill to relieve the conditions described in this chapter. In the grand scheme of things, these conditions are mosquito bites in relation to the other issues that women face during and after menopause. But these conditions are really annoying, and they vex our vanity, so you may like to know why they happen and what you can do about them. That's what this chapter is about.

Getting the Skinny on Skin

Marcia, who co-writes this book, works out regularly. Her motivation is a vivid memory of a teacher's flabby upper arm swinging back and forth as she wrote assignments on the blackboard. Marcia recalls thirty children snickering as the wobble of loose flesh seemed to move to a rhythm all its own.

The fear of children snickering at her arms has kept Marcia jogging and lifting weights on a daily basis. But she'll never forget the time she looked down as she was running to see the top of her *forearm* jiggling. Oh, the horror! What was happening? There's no fat there! As Marcia looks at her arm more closely, she realises that it isn't fat that is jiggling but her *skin!* Her skin is no longer tight on her arms: Her skin is loose to the point that it wobbles as she runs. Fortunately, Marcia's vision is so bad now that, if she doesn't wear her glasses when she runs, she doesn't see the sagging skin jiggle.

Usually, during perimenopause (the years leading up to menopause) and menopause, you're on a heightened state of alert, looking for the changes you know are happening. Some of the changes include extra laugh lines or crow's feet around your eyes. You may also notice dry skin or a dry scalp, which perhaps you didn't have before.

Making the skin and hormone connection

Menopause (more specifically the associated decline of oestrogen levels) probably accelerates many of the little annoying changes that accompany ageing. But separating the skin changes due to low oestrogen from those that come as a result of being on this planet for a long time is difficult. Forty-plus years of gravity is going to contribute to sagginess. No matter whether you're a woman or a man, your skin started fighting gravity's weight the minute you sat upright. By the time you approach your seventies, you're left with jowls instead of cheeks and a 'gobbler' instead of a nice, tight neck.

Placing blame for skin woes

Oestrogen plays a role in the great skin caper. The collagen and elastin fibres that keep your skin supple, pliant, and nicely moulded to your frame slowly deteriorate as the active form of oestrogen declines. The deterioration of collagen and elastin fibres leaves room for the wrinkles. Wrinkles (creases in your skin) show up where muscles contract. For example, when you smile, several facial muscles pull tight, forming one or more lines in the skin adjacent to your mouth. With age, these lines stay behind even when you're not smiling. Other wrinkles resemble straight or branched lines finely etched all over the weakened skin. These wrinkles are also the result of the double dip of low oestrogen levels and ageing.

The fatty layer under your skin disappears over time as well, and your skin loses its flexibility, which leads to the saggy skin Marcia watches flapping on her arms as she runs. If your skin were clothes, you'd probably go to the tailor to have it taken in. (In fact, some women do go to the tailor, also known as the plastic surgeon, to have the sags nipped and tucked.)

Medical types are divided on how much blame to apportion to gravity and how much to assign to declining levels of oestrogen. Some scientists claim that skin changes are just part of ageing, but others feel that low levels of oestrogen during the years leading up to and after menopause hasten a lot of these changes in your skin.

The hormone-imbalance crowd points out that oestrogen helps to bring moisture to body tissue. Menopause causes lower levels of *oestradiol* (the active kind of oestrogen), which causes tissues and mucous membranes all over your body to act strangely. Some women, for example, develop pimples and dry skin *at the same time*.

The bottom line is that during perimenopause and menopause your skin loses its elasticity and tightness and becomes thinner and saggier. As the fatty layer under your skin thins out over time, it is easier to see your blood vessels and you bruise more easily. Because your skin is less pliant, it tears more easily than it used to – so you may encounter more minor cuts and scrapes.

The skin-maintenance process also slows down as part of the normal ageing process in both men and women, so your body doesn't regenerate skin as quickly as it used to – another reason why you may bruise and cut more easily and heal more slowly.

Slowing down the process

Whether oestrogen treatment is effective in slowing down the skin-ageing process in menopausal women is still debatable – especially because some experts don't believe that shifting hormones have anything to do with skin changes in the first place. Experts occupy both sides of the fence on this subject.

If you want to try an oestrogen treatment, skin creams (call them *transdermal oestradiol therapies* if you're feeling knowledgeable) are more effective than oral oestrogen in preserving skin collagen. But don't get overly optimistic about the results. When you see those smiling, wrinkle-free faces on the oestrogen-cream advertisements, those women probably don't get their smooth skin, big breasts, and girlish figures from the oestrogen skin cream – rather, the lighting and air-brushing do the trick.

Although manufacturers love us to believe that face creams can hold back the ravages of time, they mostly only soften fine lines and wrinkles.

Working on wrinkles

Nothing prevents wrinkles like staying out of the sun. But if the damage is already done, you can check out products that claim to retard the wrinkling process:

✔ **Retinoid creams:** These products often use the terms *retinoic acid* and *tretinoin* and are derived from vitamin A. In fact, retinoids are vitamin A acids. Retinoid creams work by smoothing out skin pigmentation (colour), reducing brown spots and wrinkles, and giving your skin a rosy appearance. Usually, you need to use the cream for several months before you notice any improvement. Weak versions are available in over-the-counter creams but stronger versions are only available on prescription.

Some people think that because retinoids are vitamin A in disguise, they can just take mega-doses of vitamin A to improve their skin. Doing so doesn't work, however, because vitamin A is toxic in high doses and is harmful to your health.

✔ **Alpha-hydroxy creams:** Alpha-hydroxy acids work like a skin peel, removing surface skin cells. After these skin cells are removed, your skin looks rosier and smoother. Some advertisers claim that alpha-hydroxy helps your skin to produce collagen and elastin. If these claims were true, alpha-hydroxy would actually improve the layers under the skin (filling in the wrinkles from the inside out). Unfortunately, these alpha-hydroxy creams actually work from the outside in, removing old skin cells and giving your face a glow. Some of the side effects of alpha-hydroxy creams include burning, itching, and general skin pain. Newer products that contain beta-hydroxy acids incorporate a mild aspirin-like substance into the product, which is supposed to eliminate skin irritation.

✔ **Botox:** Here's one of the newer wrinkle killers. Wrinkles are caused by contraction of facial muscles (as we discuss in the section 'Making the skin and hormone connection' earlier in this chapter). Botox, a purified form of the botulism toxin, is injected into the facial muscles. It temporarily removes the wrinkle because the toxin temporarily paralyses or weakens the affected muscles. When the muscles relax, the wrinkle disappears. Botox treatments usually last for several months before the paralysis wears off and the wrinkle returns.

Shining a light on the sun's dangers

The sun is public enemy number one for your skin. Sun exposure can lead to wrinkles in your twenties or early thirties and cause your skin to go leathery and unevenly coloured years before perimenopause.

Reining in UV rays

The sun's *ultraviolet (UV) rays* inflict the greatest harm on your skin. UV rays from the sun destroy collagen fibres. The collagen fibres hold your skin tight and keep it from sagging and wrinkling. Your skin has a normal maintenance process in which old skin is sloughed off and new skin is rebuilt. UV radiation messes up this process so that the collagen fibres become disorganised and form 'solar scars'. Just 5–15 minutes of sunbathing for a fair- to moderate-skinned person can stop the skin-maintenance process for a week. UV radiation from the sun also leads to a build-up of a substance that causes the skin to stretch (*abnormal elastin*).

Caring about skin cancer

UV radiation can cause skin cancer – a serious side effect of too much sun. Skin cancer can show up years after long-term exposure to the sun.

By the time you're menopausal, your risk of skin cancer is higher because you've exposed your skin to UV radiation for quite a few years. *Malignant melanoma* is a rather rare but deadly form of skin cancer. It's most commonly diagnosed in people in their early fifties.

When you're in the sun for too long, the sun's UV radiation penetrates your skin and gets down into the DNA inside the skin cells. The UV radiation zaps and damages your DNA – serious stuff, because cell reproduction is based on DNA. Any mistakes in your DNA can have serious ramifications down the line. Sometimes, genetic mutations produce cancerous skin tumours. UV rays also suppress your skin's immune system, leaving your skin susceptible to cancer cells.

Preventing premature skin ageing

If you worry about the appearance of your skin, you're probably wondering how you can combat the skin changes that accompany the ageing process and menopause. Here are a couple of ways to keep your skin looking youthful and firm for as long as you can:

- ✔ **Don't smoke:** On average, smokers have thinner skin and more wrinkles than non-smokers. A heavy smoker is five times more likely to have a wrinkled face than a non-smoker of the same age. A 40-year-old, heavy smoker has the face of a non-smoking 60-year-old in terms of wrinkles.

- ✔ **Avoid exposure to the sun:** Exposure to ultraviolet (UV) radiation accounts for 90 per cent of the symptoms of premature skin ageing. UV radiation's also the most significant cause of skin cancers.

Sniffing Out Nasal Changes

During perimenopause and menopause, sinus problems hit some women who never had them before. Lower levels of oestrogen dry out the mucous membranes in the sinus cavities and nasal passages. Your mucous membranes are supposed to clean out foreign particles from your sinuses and nose. When the membranes are dry they can't do their job, and so your sinuses and nose become inflamed and you develop a case of *chronic rhinitis*. Most people refer to this condition with a much less scientific name – a runny nose.

To fix the problem of dryness, instead of using antihistamines or decongestants, which dry you up further, use a saline (salt) nasal spray (from a pharmacy) to moisten your mucous tissues and help them to work more effectively. Steam baths and hormone replacement therapy (HRT) also can help relieve the dryness. (See Chapter 15 for more on hormone replacement therapy (HRT).)

Handling Hairy Issues

Grey hair has nothing to do with menopause, except that both tend to occur in women over the age of 40. But menopause does bring about changes in hair patterns in ways you may never have imagined, including losing hair on your head and gaining it on your face.

These chin hairs are easily removed using tweezers or a depilatory cream, which dissolves them away. Don't shave with a razor unless you enjoy the feel of the resulting stubble regrowth.

Hair follicles are receptive to hormones. Female hormone (oestrogen) levels decrease faster than male hormone (androgen) levels, so where you once had very high levels of active oestrogen and very low levels of androgen, you now have low levels of androgen but much lower levels of active oestrogen. These lower levels of oestrogen aren't enough to block the effects of the androgen.

About one-third of women between the ages of 40 and 80 find their hair thinning all over their scalp but more so on the crown of the head. This is called *female-pattern baldness*. The amount of hair loss varies from woman to woman.

Some women have success with minoxidil solution, the same treatment recommended for balding men. Minoxidil is better at preserving hair than retrieving what was lost, so if you want to try this treatment, best to seek help sooner rather than later.

The hormonal imbalance may also cause you to grow a few hairs on your chin and other spots on your face. Hormone replacement therapy helps restore some of the balance between hormones in your body, thus helping to preserve your hair (on your head) and protect your chin from hair growth (see Chapter 15).

Chapter 8

Spicing Up Your Sex Life

. . . .

In This Chapter

▶ Understanding how your libido can cha-cha-cha while your hormones do the rumba

▶ Warming up the sheets

▶ Checking out your fertility

▶ Facing the challenges of fertility in your forties

. . . .

*F*riends of a merry widow who is dating again often ask, 'Why does anyone want sex at that age?' And when the merry widow brags, 'Sex is even better after the menopause,' her more jealous friends scoff, 'Any sex is better than what she's used to.' Some folks interpret the merry widow as putting too positive a spin on the change, but rest assured – more people continue having sex after sixty than give it up. In fact, you may enjoy the experience more as you are no longer concerned about getting pregnant or having the kids burst in at any moment.

You may decide you finally want to give those organs a work out, just as they're preparing for retirement. Or you may discover your organs are still willing, but your hormones are not. Although getting pregnant at 40 isn't impossible, and does happen, you will find it more difficult than for a woman in her twenties.

There's no question that sex changes after menopause – your changing hormones change your breasts and vagina as well as your emotional parts. But those changes don't mean the elimination of your sex life. In this chapter we tell you why and cover all the issues pertaining to sex for enjoyment and sex for reproduction as you approach, enter, and pass menopause.

Looking at Menopause and Your Libido

Menopause opens a new chapter in your life, so you shouldn't be surprised that the sexual part of your life changes. For many women, the changes are for the better. For example, even though having sex during a menstrual period is not wrong, many women refrain from sex on those days; once those menstrual periods hit the road, you have more opportunities for sex. And remember how you always get your period when on vacation, no matter how well you plan? Now you can play around to your heart's content without a visit from 'the curse'. The crankiness, cramps, and headaches that ebb and flow with your menstrual cycle now level out into a kinder and gentler expression of you.

Your libido – the desire to have sex – declines with age. Most scientific studies show little change in sexual activity between the ages of 45 and 55 years; but between 55 and 65 years, your sexual activity slows.

Although women in their sixties don't engage in sex as often as they did in their younger days, no change occurs in the frequency of orgasm or the level of sexual enjoyment. So, you may not do it as often, but sex is just as satisfying. (An interesting note: Research shows that activity with sexual partners often slows down long before women discontinue masturbating.)

The fluctuating hormones that characterise menopause and perimenopause definitely have an effect on your sex drive. Be prepared for a gradual increase or a gradual decrease in your libido. Of course, you may not notice any changes at all, but most menopausal women experience at least brief periods of higher- or lower-than-usual sex drive.

Letting your feelings act as a guide

No one knows your body better than you, so pay attention to it. Because every woman experiences menopause a little differently, learn to trust yourself.

The advice on trusting yourself should come in a double dose for changes in your *libido*. Many doctors ignore sexual issues when treating perimenopausal and menopausal women. So remember to raise the issue if your doctor doesn't.

For some helpful hints for talking to your doctor, see Chapter 6.

You can fix a drop in sexual desire in many ways. If your doctor confirms that your health is OK, you may want to consult a sex therapist (perhaps one of those available through Relate, which we list in the Resources section at the end of this book). A sex therapist can help you if your problems are behavioural or psychological in nature.

Turning up the heat

More than half of all menopausal women maintain the same level of sexual interest after menopause as before. In fact, you often feel less inhibited when the possibility of pregnancy no longer looms over your bed. Once you can safely put away your contraceptive devices, you're more free to express yourself sexually. Many women report feeling greater sexual creativity and freedom after the change. And many women who experience a mid-life divorce find that sex with a new partner (after menopause) is better than ever.

Researchers have shown the world that sexual *appetite* is not tied to oestrogen levels (although you may need some lubricant to make sex comfortable after oestrogen declines). It's really the *androgens* (male sex hormones like testosterone) made in your ovaries throughout your life that keep your sex drive running. Even after menopause (when your ovaries are out of the oestradiol-and progesterone-production game), your ovaries keep on producing androgens.

If you have sex with more than one partner during or after menopause, you still need to practise safe sex to avoid picking up a sexually transmitted infection, including HIV (human immunodeficiency virus).

Even though men don't go through a menopause as such, their testosterone levels gradually decline after the age of 40. The physiological changes don't happen overnight. Over time, men notice that it takes longer for them to get an erection and they aren't as easily aroused, which is good news for a woman who enjoys foreplay. Women whose partners suffer premature ejaculation can rejoice: That problem goes away and men gain staying power as they age.

Even if you're having fewer periods (or perhaps haven't seen one in months), don't give up your birth control until you are period-free for a full year (assuming that takes you over the age of 50 years; if you're still under 50 after one year of no periods, continue with contraception for two years after your last period). During perimenopause, your hormone levels and the chance of ovulation are wildly unpredictable. Unlikely it may be, but you may have a hormonally hot month and wind up pregnant.

Dealing with a lowered libido

A healthy self-image and adult lifestyle generally include satisfying and safe sexual activity. Yet many women are frustrated with a declining desire for sex during and after menopause. An active sex life may be important to both you and your partner. Understanding the biology behind your declining libido can help you to reach a solution.

Your sex drive can decline sooner than is desirable for several reasons. Some of these reasons are emotional – if your self-esteem declines because of changes in your life or in your body (such as weight gain), you may have to address that issue before you regain your old libido. Some of the reasons are physical – for example, painful sex is nothing to look forward to. And some of the reasons are hormonal – your hormones are changing, and to maintain your sex drive you may need to balance those hormones.

Communicating with your doctor and your partner is critical in overcoming decreased libido.

Adjusting your attitude

If you're depressed, you may have difficulty feeling amorous. Menopause in itself doesn't make you depressed, but think about the things happening during these years:

- ✔ Your kids leave home.
- ✔ Your parents age and need more attention.
- ✔ You and/or your partner retire.

Add to these challenges the everyday issues of maintaining a happy relationship and just coping in a fast-paced world. Now, the one thing that used to be reliable, your body, is also changing at a faster pace than normal. Is it any wonder that sex is the last thing on your mind?

If the lack of physical spark bothers you, you need to get rid of your emotional stressors before your libido can kick in. You may need to allocate more time to yourself. Take some time to get an exercise programme off the ground or walk regularly by yourself or with a friend to reduce your stress. Talk with friends, a therapist, your hairdresser, or minister about your challenges. And remember to bring up your anxiety or depression when you talk to your doctor.

Making sure that sex isn't a hurtin' thing

Hormonal changes can cause your vaginal lining to thin, making it more fragile and susceptible to tearing. Your vaginal lining also produces less lubrication. Your vagina becomes more delicate and tender. Vaginal connective tissues are also less pliant and your nerve endings more sensitive.

The result of this biological shuffle is that intercourse is often painful. Sexual activity that used to deliver great pleasure now causes pain instead. The thought of this discomfort may make you prefer a headache or clearing out your sock drawer when your partner makes amorous advances, but all is not lost. You can alleviate painful intercourse in a variety of ways:

✔ **Maintain an active sex life.** Regular sexual activity keeps blood circulating in your vulva and slows the drying process. So maintaining an active sex life helps postpone or avoid the pain associated with dry vaginal tissues.

✔ **Talk to your partner about the more sensitive you.** Most men aren't aware that hormonal changes affect your vulva and vagina. Explain to your partner that the two of you need to figure out new bedroom strategies that are mutually satisfying.

✔ **Use a lubricant during intercourse to help keep things moving.** Lubricants can afford hours of interpersonal pleasure. Some women and their partners make lubricant application a part of foreplay. Check lubricants are water-based if you use latex condoms or a diaphragm.

Sometimes, women experience regular discomfort due to vaginal dryness – not just during sex. If you're one of these women, you can use other types of lubricants on a regular basis to relieve this irritation. (Check out Chapter 6 on tips for dealing with vaginal dryness.)

Don't use oestrogen cream as a sexual lubricant. You partner can absorb the oestrogen cream, which can lead to problems; at least one case of breast cancer in a man is possibly due to his wife using vaginal oestrogen cream as a lubricant.

Talking about Testosterone

Don't forget that men, as well as women, experience declining libido as they age. If you're noticing changes in your sexual relationship, remember that your partner's hormones are changing, too. Men produce much more testosterone than women, but when they reach 40, their testosterone levels start declining. However, most men don't notice an appreciable change in their libido for about another 10 years. Around the age of 50 or so, the drop in testosterone causes men to stop having *psychogenic erections* (erections from just thinking about sex), and men who are used to getting an erection at the drop of a hat have a bit more difficulty getting things moving.

So, if you're worried because your partner isn't pursuing you like he used to, your menopause is probably not at the heart of the matter. Your partner is probably experiencing hormonal changes of his own, even though his change isn't as dramatic as yours.

Keeping Sex Sexy

If you notice changes in your sexual relationship, work with your partner to make things better. Your relationship can evolve to a new level of meaning and pleasure.

First, you need to communicate with your partner and take stock of your situation. Is it a libido thing for you? Is it a libido thing for him? Is it technique? Is it timing? You need to find out what's going on.

As you and your partner get older and both your testosterone levels decline, try spending more time on foreplay. You may both need more stimulation before intercourse. You may also need to incorporate lubricants into your foreplay if you have vaginal dryness.

Try some different techniques to provide enough stimulation for your man to get an erection. Hand stimulation or oral sex may get him started. You can also turn to books and counsellors. Or visit Amora, the Academy of Sex and Relationships in London `www.amoralondon.com` for an exciting and inspiring look at human sexuality and how to improve your love life.

Although you may come from the sex, booze, and drugs generation, these words no longer work together. Take a look at some of the things that can douse your flame:

- ✔ **Alcohol:** One drink may help you relax and feel less inhibited, but several drinks can put a damper on your libido, arousal, performance, and ability to reach orgasm.

- ✔ **Prescription drugs:** Serotonin boosters, antidepressants, blood pressure pills, sleeping pills, and many other drugs frequently prescribed for women over 50 can take a toll on your libido. Remind your doctor about what medications you take when you discuss your libido and sexual performance. Your doctor can usually switch you to other medications that don't affect your sex drive.

- ✔ **Tobacco:** The nicotine in cigarettes and other tobacco products constricts blood vessels making it more difficult for blood to rush to your sexual organs. You then find arousal more difficult and experiencing a satisfactory conclusion harder still.

Diabetes and other medical problems also cause loss of sexual desire and performance problems. Always tell your doctor about changes in your libido because they can result from other medical conditions.

Don't blame the oestrogen!

Although scientists have found no evidence linking changes in oestrogen levels to a declining libido, the *balance* between oestrogen and testosterone is thought to make a difference.

This subject is a bit controversial so here's both sides of the argument. On one side are scientists who conclude that supplementing your testosterone during menopause increases your libido. On the other side are the researchers who believe that prescribing testosterone is neither safe nor effective for women who complain of low libido.

Testosterone is produced naturally in your ovaries and has a positive impact on your libido, mood, vitality, sense of wellbeing, bone, and muscle. But, even before menopause, your body slows down its production of testosterone. After menopause, you produce only half as much testosterone as you do during your reproductive years. So your libido declines if your testosterone levels are too low.

You don't want too much testosterone either, however, as testosterone can promote breast and liver cancer. Plus, too much testosterone

relative to oestrogen can unleash the effects of testosterone that oestrogen keeps under control, such as facial hair, increased libido, redistribution of body fat (it moves to the middle of your body), and acne.

Some doctors shy away from prescribing testosterone as part of hormone replacement therapy (HRT) because they're afraid of upsetting your oestrogen/testosterone balance and causing unpleasant side effects. The trick for the doctor is to keep your testosterone levels high enough to avoid one set of side effects (including low libido) and in balance with your other hormones to avoid another set of side effects (facial hair or acne, for example). You are therefore started on a low dose initially and this is only increased if necessary.

Scientists who view testosterone as a worthy treatment for libido problems believe that the side effects are due to excessively high dosages. Proponents of testosterone suggest using very low dosages and maintaining a balance between the levels of testosterone and oestrogen.

Focusing on Fertility and Beyond

The hormone dance that ends in menopause actually begins years before you stop having periods. Most women don't know what time the ball begins and are shocked when they have trouble getting pregnant in their thirties.

Your fertility begins to decline in your late twenties. Women in their early to mid-twenties have only a fifty/fifty chance of becoming pregnant each cycle, even if they have intercourse during the peak time for conception. In your late twenties to early thirties that chance drops to 40 per cent each cycle, and by your late thirties your chance of getting pregnant is less than 30 per cent. Figure 8-1 shows the odds per cycle.

Men start to lose their fertility in their thirties. So, if you're in your late thirties and your partner is five years older than you, your chances of becoming pregnant in any given cycle may drop to 20 per cent. This means that, on average, you have to try for more cycles to get pregnant. You can still conceive if you're in your late thirties, but on average you need a few months more than a younger woman, especially if your partner is older than you.

Figure 8-1: Percentage of pregnancies achieved by women trying for a baby, per menstrual cycle by age.

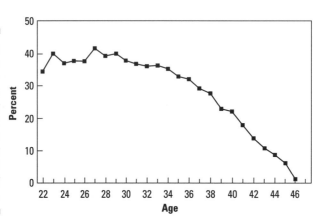

Many women who put off motherhood until their late thirties need help to get pregnant. Read on to discover what fertility treatment is all about.

Evaluating whether you're too late to start a family

When you are a teenager, your parents, teachers, and friends warn that practically all you have to do to get pregnant is to jump in a swimming pool with a boy. A slight exaggeration maybe, but generally getting pregnant is easier in your teens than in your thirties.

Doctors describe women who find it difficult getting pregnant as *infertile*. *Infertility* is usually defined as the inability to get pregnant after trying for one year.

Getting a head start on pregnancy

To optimise your chances of pregnancy, here are some things you can work on before you see your doctor:

✔ Ensure that your diet is healthy – try to eat at least five portions of fruit and veg each day.

✔ Exercise regularly.

✔ Plan your sexual activities so you have intercourse several times during your ovulation cycle (see the sidebar 'Figuring out when you're fertile' for more on your ovulation cycle).

✔ Rid your life of as much stress as you can. Go on holiday, get plenty of rest, and try to stay on an even keel emotionally.

Knowing when you're fertile

You're most fertile right before and during ovulation. Some women can tell when they ovulate because they feel a dull pain in the area of their ovary. But such insight is a rare talent, and most women need to employ a trick or two. The simplest and cheapest test involves taking your temperature (check out the sidebar 'Figuring out when you're fertile' for more details on this). Using temperature charts is an accurate ovulation test, but you have to stick with the process and take your temperature every day, beginning on the first day of your period. Also, you only find out that you've ovulated after the fact. Figure 8-2 shows a sample ovulation chart.

An easier way to know whether you're ovulating is to use an ovulation predictor test available from supermarkets and pharmacies. Ovulation predictor tests are easy to use.

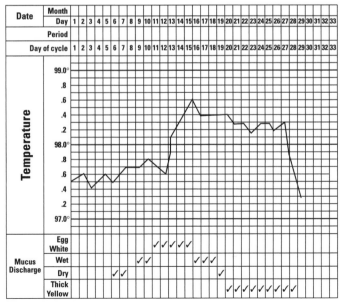

Figure 8-2: One woman's record of her fertility cycle.

When you ovulate, the *follicle* (the little sac that holds the egg) in your ovary releases an egg. The egg begins its journey down your fallopian tube and into your uterus. The egg lives for only 6–24 hours after ovulation. Because sperm can live for two to seven days inside you (if you have good, fertility-friendly mucus), having sex just before and during ovulation is the best way to get pregnant. Men can make about 50,000 sperm a minute, but it takes only one to make a baby.

Tracing the yin and yang of conception

Many things have to happen correctly to make a baby:

- ✔ Your ovaries must produce follicles.
- ✔ The follicles have to grow big enough to release an egg.
- ✔ You need the right hormone balance to release the egg and for the egg to survive its journey.
- ✔ You need clear fallopian tubes with no obstructions so that the egg can travel all the way to your uterus to meet some sperm.
- ✔ Your hormones must create the right environment for the egg to be fertilised and nestle comfortably into the lining of your uterus.

Out-of-whack hormones are to blame for most infertility problems in peri-menopausal women.

Facing up to potential problems

In this section we look at some of the common things that go wrong during attempts to conceive and ways to tackle these problems:

- ✔ **Problem:** Your ovaries aren't producing follicles or the follicles don't get big enough to produce an egg because your hormones are out of balance.

  Medical tests: Your doctor is likely to perform a series of blood tests at several points throughout your cycle to determine whether your hormones are at the right levels to produce follicles, ovulate, and provide safe harbour for a fertilised egg in your uterus. If all is well with your hormones, your doctor may take a peak at your ovaries using a sonogram (ultrasound) at about the midway point of your cycle to see whether you're making healthy follicles and whether your follicles are growing to a healthy size. Checking your progesterone level on day 21 shows whether you're still ovulating.

  Solution: Your doctor may suggest fertility medications to help you produce more follicles.

✔ **Problem:** Your fallopian tubes are obstructed, so the egg can't reach your uterus.

Medical tests: Your doctor may do a *laparoscopy* to look at your tubes to see whether they are clear and examine your other organs to see whether they are diseased. Another common test is called a *hysterosalpingogram* – your doctor injects a dye and takes an X-ray of your fallopian tubes and uterus to see whether your tubes are open and your uterus in good shape.

Solutions: Sometimes the test finds evidence of endometriosis, a condition in which womb lining cells travel to the pelvis to cause inflammation. Your doctor may treat endometriosis with surgery or medication.

✔ **Problem:** The *endometrium* (the lining of your uterus) may not thicken enough for a fertilised egg to latch on and snuggle in.

Medical test: Your doctor may do an *endometrial biopsy* to rule out a hormonal deficiency. If you are low on progesterone, your endometrium doesn't get thick enough for a fertilised egg to nestle in.

Solution: Your doctor may put you on a hormone regimen of progesterone after ovulation.

If you and your partner seek professional help with fertility, both of you are tested and treatment depends on those initial tests. A normal series of semen tests suggests you need further investigations, while an abnormal series of semen tests suggests your partner needs further assessment.

Taking a dipstick to your oestrogen

When you seek assistance in your bid to get pregnant, one of the first things your fertility doctor does is check whether you're capable of ovulating. In order to ovulate, you need both the right kind of oestrogen and the right amount of this particular form of oestrogen in your bloodstream. This form of oestrogen is called *oestradiol*. Your doctor will probably take a blood sample to check your oestradiol.

As you approach menopause, your body produces less oestradiol but continues to produce oestrone. When it comes to producing follicles and ovulating, oestradiol is the kind that counts: Without adequate levels of oestradiol, your ovaries don't produce eggs. By measuring both types of oestrogen, your doctor can see whether you're heading toward menopause or whether you have other hormonal problems. (See Chapter 2 for more on the different types of hormones women produce.)

Because your hormone levels fluctuate during perimenopause, you may still have periods but you may not ovulate each month. Your oestradiol levels may be high one month but low another month. Some months are good for getting pregnant and some months are not so good. By measuring your oestradiol levels each month, your doctor can see whether this is a good month for producing an egg.

Messing up the nest with hormones

Sometimes hormonal problems occur after the follicle releases the egg. Normally the follicle pops open to release the egg and then hangs around long enough to produce progesterone (after the follicle releases the egg, the empty sac is called a *corpus luteum*). The corpus luteum eventually disintegrates.

Progesterone production is necessary for thickening the uterine lining and preparing it for the egg. If the follicle doesn't produce enough progesterone, problems arise that can put an end to conception. If the lining isn't ready, the fertilised egg won't nestle into your endometrium properly.

Progesterone production slows down during perimenopause and menopause, so you may have problems making a home for a fertilised egg.

Understanding that periods don't mean you're fertile

Even in your prime baby-conceiving years, you need everything aligned properly to get pregnant. But as you move into your perimenopausal years, some months you ovulate and some months you don't. As time goes on, you experience more and more cycles in which you don't ovulate.

You may have a period even if you don't ovulate.

Getting pregnant outside the bedroom

Couples have trouble getting pregnant for many reasons. The reasons described in this chapter are some of the more common problems due to hormonal imbalances in perimenopausal women.

A full coverage of fertility treatments would take another complete book, so we just hit a few of the highlights here. If you're past your prime in terms of the fertility game, today's fertility clinics have a host of conception alternatives outside the bedroom. Your chances of getting pregnant depend on your individual circumstances, but some fertility clinics have conception rates that are higher than others.

If you have ethical or religious concerns about artificial reproductive therapy, these options may not suit you.

Here are some of the fertility techniques in use today:

Al: Artificial insemination

If the reproduction problems you're experiencing relate to your partner's sperm, you may want to consider artificial insemination. In artificial insemination, your doctor places semen into your uterus or vaginal canal using a tiny tube. Think of this procedure as a head start for the backstroke-challenged sperm.

Mother's little helper: In vitro fertilisation

If you're having problems conceiving, another alternative is *in vitro* fertilisation (IVF). In this procedure, your doctor gives you medication to stimulate your ovaries to produce several eggs – three to ten eggs in a cycle (compared with just one or two, which you normally produce per cycle). When the eggs are mature, the doctor suctions the eggs out of your ovaries. Your partner produces a semen specimen to fertilise the eggs. (Fresh ejaculate is best, but frozen sperm and even sperm from a donor may also do the trick.) The doctor takes the sperm, mixes it with the eggs, and tucks the dish containing the sperm and eggs into an incubator. After a few days, the doctor checks the dish to see whether any of the eggs have been fertilised. With luck, one or more have been fertilised and the doctor replants one embryo into your body. Then you wait to see whether the embryo latches on to the lining of your uterus, making you pregnant.

In vitro fertilisation has no guarantees. The procedure is expensive and has risks. The medication may increase your future risk of cancer of the ovary, and your ovaries may over-stimulate to produce several follicles, which is uncomfortable due to pressure pain. Finally, you may have great success in producing lots of eggs and producing multiple embryos: The risk to the lives and health of mother and babies go up astronomically when more than two or three babies are in the womb.

Taking the good with the bad

We have good news and bad news regarding conception. We don't want you walking away from this chapter on a down note, so we start this section with a few gloomy stats and then turn our attention to the good stuff.

When you hit the age of about 35–38 (some experts say as early as 30), your fertility gradually declines. Your fertility drops precipitously at age 40. Unfortunately, around this time, your risk of spontaneous miscarriage starts to rise. By age 45, you have a fifty/fifty chance of suffering a spontaneous miscarriage if you conceive. Also, by the time you reach 45, the risk of chromosomal abnormalities in the baby increases to 1 chance in 40. In other words, for every 40 babies conceived in women aged 45 and older, one baby has a chromosomal abnormality such as Down's syndrome or spina bifida.

However, becoming a mum for the first time after 40 also has advantages. For example, the perimenopausal symptom of interrupted sleep means you're probably already awake when your baby cries. You and your newborn are on the same wavelength, and you have someone to talk to when you wake up.

If you have waited to have a family, you are probably better prepared than much younger women for the sacrifices you need to make to nurture your children. You may be in a much better position to devote your time and attention to your children compared with women in their twenties. Establishing careers, entertaining friends, travelling, and other interests often preoccupy life during your twenties and thirties. Now perhaps you're more willing to make time to raise a family.

Chapter 9

Thinking through Mental and Emotional Issues

---

*M*any of us have 'senior moments' even before menopause – those times when you forget how to spell simple words such as *apple* or you go to introduce a friend you've known for years and forget her name. Or maybe you find yourself spending more time thinking 'What did I come in here for?'

You're not alone. Many women experience these mental lapses during perimenopause and menopause. Some women even experience this type of forgetfulness long before menopause – during their menstrual cycle when oestrogen levels are at their lowest. The forgetfulness is because oestrogen plays a major role in memory functions.

Some perimenopausal and menopausal women also fall prey to emotional slumps. Some of these slumps are due to fluctuating hormone levels that prompt emotional moments (remember your moody adolescent years?), while others are an understandable reaction to the symptoms you're dealing with and the stage of your life.

Not all women experience mental and emotional problems during perimenopause or menopause. Like premenstrual syndrome (PMS), these symptoms are more severe in some women than others, depending on how sensitive you are to hormonal swings. If you have a history of memory lapses and heightened emotions in connection with your menstrual cycle, you're likely to experience them in perimenopausal and menopausal too.

In this chapter, we cover some of the emotional and memory symptoms you may experience, how they're related to your hormones, and how to tell whether a symptom is hormonal or psychological.

Understanding the Mental and Emotional Stresses of Menopause

Fortunately, with 40 or 50 years of emotional experience behind you, you're quite prepared to cope with the challenges life throws your way. Mid-life changes present you with openings – and you can view openings as voids (negative) or as opportunities for new experiences (positive). And research has shown that people who have a positive outlook on life are likely to live longer and in better health than those who think negatively.

If emotional issues or mental lapses bother you during these years, visit your doctor. Life events may trigger temporary mental or emotional issues, but a temporary mental state is quite different from a debilitating condition. If your emotional state severely interferes with your daily life for a prolonged period of time, your doctor can assess whether you have a depressive illness and whether you may benefit from antidepressant drugs or a referral for counselling.

Many physical conditions can lead to mental and emotional problems – and menopause is certainly one of these conditions.

The medical establishment didn't accept hot flushes as an actual physical condition (as opposed to whining) until the late 1970s, so you may not be surprised to hear that doctors sometimes forget to take hormones into consideration when you experience mental or emotional symptoms. Even if you ask 'Do you think that it is related to menopause?' your doctor may say, 'You're too young for the menopause', or 'No, because you're still having periods.'

You may have to take the initiative and educate your medical advisor: Symptoms due to oestrogen fluctuations are at least as common in peri-menopause as they are during menopause itself. You may have to insist on a test to check your hormone levels. And if you meet resistance, ask your friends for the name of a more receptive doctor.

You have oestrogen receptors all over your brain, particularly in areas associated with memory and mood, because your brain needs oestrogen to function properly. So, a fall in your oestrogen levels can affect your mental and emotional health.

You may experience some of the mental and emotional symptoms associated with menopause during your regular menstrual cycle. Hormone levels shift throughout the menstrual cycle, so you have a few low-oestrogen days just before starting your period (see Chapter 2 for details on your hormone rhythms).

If you are familiar with those three little letters – PMS (premenstrual syndrome) – your PMS symptoms may be an appetiser for the main course. Memory lapses, fuzzy thinking, depression, anxiety, and mood swings – all those memories from your youth – may come calling for a longer visit during perimenopause and menopause. And no, you can't turn off the lights and pretend you're not at home like you do when family members show up unannounced.

Separating Menopausal Symptoms from Psychological Disorders

The mental and emotional changes you may experience during perimenopause and menopause are different from those that can accompany psychological disorders. For example, going through bouts of depression isn't unusual during perimenopause and menopause. So how do you know whether you're heading for a depressive illness or whether your symptoms are related to your menopause?

During your younger days, you may remember feeling moody or blue for a few days each month before your period. But most women in their forties and fifties experience these changes at the same time as they're dealing with other life-changing events such as their parents ageing, the death of a loved one, marital problems, an empty nest, retirement, and job loss.

Everyone feels sad, dejected, or blue now and then. You may feel upset when you look in the mirror and see a woman who has a few more wrinkles today than last year and who still hasn't won the Nobel Prize. Or perhaps you are in the midst of profound mourning after the death of a loved one. Such sorrow may last for several months – which is a completely normal grieving response to a deeply felt emotional loss. The major difference between sad feelings and a true major depressive illness is that sad feelings eventually pass – but depression doesn't.

Depression envelops you in a sort of psychic cloud, numbing you with thoughts of a bleak outlook that never changes. A psychological disorder such as depression interferes with your sleep, appetite, sexual interest, self-image, and attitude. Herein lies the problem of determining whether you're experiencing depression or perimenopausal/menopausal symptoms – the hormonal changes also interfere with your sleep, mood, and libido. But when you don't snap out of your dark mood – the cloud doesn't lift after weeks, months or, if left untreated, even years – you move into the category of psychological disorder.

You typically experience symptoms of menopause over a limited period of time, in episodes that come and go as your hormone levels fluctuate. Although your loved ones may disagree, these symptoms don't completely alter your everyday life. Your symptoms may make you unpleasant to know sometimes, but they're not debilitating.

The mental and emotional changes that you experience because of hormonal changes shouldn't interfere with your daily life, damage your friendships or relationships with work colleagues, leave you feeling unable to manage your normal schedule of activities, or prompt you to use alcohol or drugs to help you feel better. If your symptoms do provoke changes such as these, seek medical help before your low mood spirals out of control.

Dealing With the Head Games

Your memory works because *neurons* (nerve cells) communicate with each other via neural connectors. In everyday life, neurons and neural connectors are damaged over time. A decrease in oestrogen can also cause problems because your brain needs the stimulation of oestrogen to build more neural connectors.

The mind games associated with menopause are tricky and come on gradually – so gradually that you may be unsure whether your feelings are normal for you or whether they are something new. You may think that you're going crazy. Your brain just doesn't seem to work the way it used to. Some of the symptoms you may experience include the following:

- **Fuzzy thinking:** Having trouble staying focused at work? Do you feel like you're walking around in a fog some days? Many women complain of problems concentrating during perimenopause and menopause. A shortened attention span is also associated with hormonal change.

- **Headaches:** Some women who experience migraines during their menstrual cycles lose them after menopause. Other women first have migraines or have worse migraines during menopause.

  More women than men get migraines. Migraine headaches generally start after puberty, which may indicate a connection to female sex hormones. But the connection is strange. Your blood vessels constrict during a migraine attack, but oestrogen helps dilate (widen) blood vessels – so you may think that the oestrogen in hormone replacement therapy (HRT) would relieve your migraines. But some women on HRT actually get worse migraines with treatment, while other women get oestrogen-withdrawal headaches from a decrease in that hormone. So, doctors still don't understand the connection between oestrogen and headaches.

✔ **Memory lapses:** Some but not all women experience memory lapses during menopause. Try to keep things in perspective, however: Losing your car keys or temporarily forgetting how to spell a simple word is aggravating, but not recognising your partner or child is another story altogether. Just because you occasionally experience the can't-find-my-pencil type of memory loss doesn't mean that you have or are likely to develop Alzheimer's disease. (See the sidebar 'Connecting oestrogen and Alzheimer's disease' for more information on Alzheimer's disease.)

Looking at the link between oestrogen and memory

Researchers still don't know all the specifics of how oestrogen helps your brain remember, but they do know that oestrogen helps build healthy connections between neurons in your brain. Oestrogen also improves blood flow to your brain by dilating and relaxing your blood vessels, so they don't develop spasms. (See Chapter 5 for more on how oestrogen keeps your blood vessels healthy.) Both of these effects of oestrogen keep your mind from going to mush.

Because oestrogen plays a big part in regulating brain function, women who take HRT seem to have fewer mental symptoms than other menopausal women. One study found that healthy menopausal women using oestrogen had better short-term memory than healthy menopausal women not taking oestrogen.

Within as little as three weeks of starting HRT, many perimenopausal women have better verbal memory, mental concentration, reasoning, and reaction times.

Your oestrogen levels must rise to a certain level to have a positive effect on memory, so make sure that your doctor evaluates your oestrogen levels by taking a blood test and then changes your HRT dose if you have no improvement in memory after treatment begins.

Beating the memory game

The least invasive (and most effective) way to improve your memory during and after menopause also improves the rest of your health: Follow a balanced diet and exercise regularly. Remember (no pun intended) that your brain needs exercise too. Whether you're 5 or 50 years old, you need to exercise your brain (we provide suggestions below) to keep your neurons active and improve your memory. Here are a few ways you can boost your memory:

✔ **Check your thyroid and ovarian hormone levels:** Your doctor may check your hormone levels to determine whether your symptoms are related to menopause or whether you may have another problem such as an underactive thyroid gland.

✔ **Don't smoke:** Among the other undesirable effects of smoking, those grey clouds suffocate your nerve cells by restricting the amount of oxygen reaching your brain.

✔ **Exercise your body:** Walk, swim, dance or practise yoga. Whatever exercise you choose, just get moving! Brisk aerobic activity, three to five times a week, for 30 minutes to an hour at a time, keeps the oxygen flowing to your brain, which improves your memory and your mood.

✔ **Get enough sleep:** Lack of oestrogen can disrupt your sleep. Whether your particular brand of sleep deprivation is due to stress, having to urinate regularly, low levels of oestrogen, or your partner's snoring, lack of sleeps affects your memory.

Take care when using sleeping pills, as they interrupt your normal sleep patterns, which in turn can have a negative impact on your memory. Ideally, your doctor should not give you sleeping pills for more than two weeks in a row. If you do need sleeping pills, try to take them only every other night, to help you get back into a normal sleep routine.

✔ **Limit your alcohol consumption:** Alcohol damages nerve cells in the brain and depletes your body of the vitamins necessary for building neural connections. Try to limit your alcohol consumption to no more than three units of alcohol per week if possible, and certainly no more than two units per day, on average.

✔ **Mobilise your mental muscle:** Do crossword puzzles, attempt Sudoku, read, take an evening class, or try memorising poems or recipes. Stimulating your brain helps you build new neural connections.

✔ **Revitalise with vitamins:** Certain vitamins help build nerve cells and the neural connectors that you need to remember things (or to just plain think). Among the more important vitamins are:

- **B vitamins:** This group includes vitamins B1, B2, B6, and B12. You can find B vitamins in meat, enriched flour, yeast extract and wheat germ.

- **Folic acid:** Folic acid is also a B vitamin but, unlike many other B vitamins, is found primarily in vegetables rather than flour and meat. Green leafy vegetables, such as spinach, spring greens, kale, and broccoli, are rich in folic acid.

Connecting oestrogen and Alzheimer's disease

When you catch yourself forgetting something, is your first thought 'Oh gosh! I'm getting Alzheimer's!'? If so, you're referring to the dementia associated with Alzheimer's disease. *Dementia* is the loss of intellectual abilities such as memory, judgement, and orientation. Alzheimer's disease is one of many causes of dementia.

Research into Alzheimer's disease is in its infancy. Scientists know that the disease damages neurons in the parts of the brain responsible for memory, speech, emotions, and thinking, but they haven't discovered why this happens.

Oestrogen appears to play a role in Alzheimer's disease. Receptors for sex hormones, such as oestrogen, progesterone, and testosterone, are located in the parts of the brain that Alzheimer's disease damages. Researchers also know that oestrogen stimulates the growth of nerve connections. One study shows that women taking hormone replacement therapy (HRT) are about half as likely to have Alzheimer's disease as women not taking HRT. In another study, women with Alzheimer's disease seem to improve slightly when put on HRT.

- **Antioxidants:** Antioxidants include vitamins A, C, and E, beta-carotene and selenium. Antioxidants work like rust protection for your cells. Oxidation of your cells has a similar effect as oxidation of metal – rust – and damages and eventually kills your cells.

Take a look at Chapter 18 to find out more about the importance of vitamins during and after menopause. Most women need a multivitamin supplement to get sufficient dosages of these vitamins.

Sorting Out the Commotion in Your Emotions

As a woman, if you're going to develop depression or an anxiety disorder in your lifetime you're most likely to do so in your late thirties or early forties. A hormonal link between depression and menopause seems to exist. Aside from this fairly obvious coincidence in timing, certain physical characteristics of women with depression point to lower levels of oestrogen as a factor: Women with depression tend to have lower oestrogen levels, and their oestrogen levels go up after they pull out of the depression. Also, women with depression have lower bone density than non-depressed women. Low bone density is another common by-product of low oestrogen levels (check out Chapter 4 for more on oestrogen and your bones).

Feeling your way through your emotional symptoms

Menopause can feel like you are on a fairground ride of emotional ups and downs. If you normally experience premenstrual symptoms (PMS), these emotional upheavals may seem familiar. If you are normally affected by hormonal swings, however, you may feel as if you are going mad. You are not. What you are experiencing is perfectly normal, expected and – thankfully – temporary. Here are some emotional changes you may notice as you approach menopause:

- **Anxiety:** You're driving along and all of a sudden you feel panicky. Anxiety causes both emotional and physical symptoms. Emotionally, you may feel irritable or have trouble focusing your mind. Physically, your heart may start beating like you're sprinting a 100-metre dash. You wonder whether you should head straight to hospital. Heart *palpitations* or a racing heart with butterflies in your stomach are common during perimenopause and menopause.

- **Depression:** If you're dealing with interrupted sleep, hot flushes, or memory lapses, avoiding depression altogether is hard. If you previously had depression linked to PMS or after childbirth (postnatal depression), you're more likely to experience depression during the change.

- **Increased sensitivity:** You may feel that life isn't fair, that everything is all your fault, or you may find yourself looking for a fight. Performing at any level that falls short of perfection can cause a negative emotional reaction. Or you may break down in tears – with or without reason.

- **Mood swings:** One minute everything is fine, and the next you're sad and gloomy. You may find it difficult dealing with family situations, relationships at home, or professional relationships.

Understanding and getting relief from your emotional symptoms

When your oestrogen levels drop, the amount of the hormone *serotonin* decreases. Serotonin helps decrease anxiety, so if you have less serotonin, you tend to get more anxious. A drop in serotonin also aggravates irritability and heart palpitations. Your doctor may prescribe serotonin-enhancing antidepressants to relieve your anxiety during perimenopause and menopause.

Selective serotonin-reuptake inhibitors (SSRIs) can come to your rescue by increasing your serotonin levels. When your brain chemicals get back in balance, you may well find relief from your symptoms of depression.

Doctors also use SSRIs to treat depression due to an imbalance between oestrogen and progesterone in your body. When your oestrogen levels are lower during perimenopause and menopause, progesterone can temporarily overpower the effects of oestrogen and testosterone in your brain, which in turn affects serotonin balance. If your serotonin is out of balance, you may feel weepy, irritable, grumpy, or downright ugly.

You may consider treating anxiety and depression with acupuncture, biofeedback, yoga, relaxation, herbal remedies, or massage. We talk about these complementary therapies in Chapter 16.

Your forties and fifties are a time of change – not only in your body but also in your everyday routines. These lifestyle changes can worsen the hormonal dance in your body.

Situational stress triggers changes in ovarian function. When your ovaries are stressed, such as during a major lifestyle change, your hormone production can drop off, causing emotional upsets. A vicious circle ensues: Certain life events cause mood swings, and the mood swings trigger changes in your internal hormones, which exaggerate the swing. So, life events may start your mental and emotional symptoms, but hormonal changes turn up the volume.

Managing Your Family

Raising children is an emotional experience. Put the whole picture in perspective: You're at mid-life, and you're juggling a host of responsibilities, including a job, childcare, household chores, a relationship with your partner, and maybe an ageing parent or in-law. No wonder you're a little scatterbrained and walking round in a fog. Caring for a family during menopause can leave you deprived of sleep, irritable, and feeling a bit moody.

Caring for ageing parents

When you hit mid-life, your parents are usually hitting their golden years. You may feel like a _sandwich generation_, – caring for ageing parents while trying to hold down the fort at home with your kids. Parenting 80-year-olds and 4-year-olds at the same time isn't unusual nowadays. The anxiety of trying to manage multiple households and meet the care needs of those closest to you is a legitimate reason for feeling guilty, inadequate, depressed, and irritable. Throw hormonal imbalance into the mix and things get really crazy. It's not just menopause; it's life, but this book offers plenty of solutions to help steer you through.

Experiencing the empty nest (or wishing your nest was empty)

When you hit menopause, perhaps your kids are leaving home, have recently left home, or *should* have left home. The house seems strangely quiet, the routines you've had for 18 or more years are interrupted, and you feel a simultaneous sense of freedom and loneliness. The world that used to revolve around school events comes to a screeching halt, creating a void and an opportunity all at the same time.

Or maybe your kids are teenagers when you reach menopause. The teenage years can fill a family with turmoil because the house is full of people whose hormones are in flux. After all, puberty has many similarities with menopause in terms of hormonal imbalances and the associated mental/emotional changes.

Some women, of course, face menopause having not had children for whatever reason, and this is just as difficult emotionally, as your fertile years draw to a close.

Retiring, gracefully or not

Ending a career is emotionally challenging. Like sending your kids off into the world after school, the abrupt shift in day-to-day routines that accompanies retirement adds stress to your life. Even if you're counting down the days until early retirement, the change can play games with your emotions. If you're used to getting your fulfilment at work, you may find your self-esteem takes a hit after retirement. How in the world are they managing without you? With extra time on your hands, you may feel unneeded.

No matter what your exact situation is, you have plenty of good reasons for a heightened emotional stage during mid-life. Hormones are not the only cause of problems during your forties and fifties. The everyday world you live in is stressful enough in itself.

If you have more time on your hands, take the opportunity to develop new interests and hobbies. Keep your mind active reading, solving puzzles, learning a foreign language or gaining new qualifications. Join clubs and volunteer for charity work to meet people and contribute to the community around you.

Part III
Treating the Effects

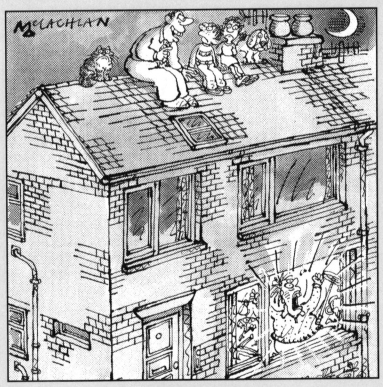

'Mummy's forgotten to pick up her HRT
tablets from the chemist.'

In this part . . .

If you're like most women, the barrage of newsflashes and special reports on hormone therapy that seem to pop up a few times a year may leave your head spinning. Flash: 'Never take hormones.' Report: 'Never stop taking hormones.' Getting a handle on the risks and benefits of hormone therapy can be challenging. In this part, we attempt to demystify the subject, so that you're in a position to make informed decisions (with the assistance of your doctor) about whether hormone therapy is right for you.

In the chapters that follow, we present you with the latest information regarding hormone therapy and its relationship to your cardiovascular system, breast cancer, your reproductive organs, and other health conditions. We also provide a load of information on non-hormonal treatments (both conventional treatments, such as medications, and non-conventional routes like herbal therapy and acupuncture) for many of the symptoms and conditions facing menopausal women.

Chapter 10

Homing in on Hormone Replacement Therapy

*H*ormone replacement therapy (HRT) is not right for everyone, but it definitely can relieve menopausal symptoms such as vaginal atrophy, hot flushes, and night sweats. HRT can also prevent or postpone osteoporosis (brittle bones) although other drugs are now preferred for this specific problem.

Some women worship HRT, some women fear it, and some women experiment with it to figure out the types, combinations, and dosages that are right for them to maximise the protective effects of HRT while minimising the risks. (Arguments about the potential risks of HRT abound, and we discuss them thoroughly in many chapters of this book, particularly Chapter 15.)

But many women aren't comfortable enough with their level of knowledge about HRT to make up their minds about where they stand on the subject. Trying to understand the full significance of the choices available is frustrating and confusing. This chapter explains the various hormones and hormone replacement therapy regimens and how they work.

Hormones are powerful, so try to understand exactly what you are putting in your body.

Defining Hormone Replacement Therapy

Some experts don't include the term 'replacement' when referring to hormone replacement therapy because 'replacement' implies that a *deficiency* exists. Producing lower levels of oestrogen hormone isn't a disease but one of many natural, normal transitions that your body goes through during your lifetime. The simpler and more accurate term for the hormones prescribed during perimenopause and menopause is *hormone therapy*. This term reflects a more progressive attitude towards the menopause. However, as the term hormone replacement therapy – or HRT – is in common use, we use the term in this book.

The types of oestrogen used in HRT are similar to natural forms of oestrogen. Synthetic versions of progesterone (known as progestogens), however, are different from natural progestogens: The synthetic versions are more stable than natural progesterone so they are more easily delivered into the body in a usable form. Unfortunately, these progestogens have more side effects than natural progesterone as they are man-made hormones.

Hormone replacement therapy (HRT) refers to the administration of oestrogen and progestogen to relieve perimenopausal and menopausal symptoms. Doctors often prescribe hormones during *perimenopause* (the years before menopause when you experience many of the symptoms associated with menopause, such as hot flushes and sleeplessness). HRT relieves *urogenital atrophy* (the thinning and drying of your vagina and lower urinary tract) exacerbated by low levels of oestrogen. For many women, the hormone boost also improves their mood and sense of wellbeing.

After menopausal symptoms have abated, however, doctors usually recommend that a woman stops taking HRT, as the UK Committee on Safety of Medicines recommends that the minimum effective dose of HRT is used for the shortest duration of time. The reason is because prolonged use of HRT increases your risk of abnormal blood clotting and stroke, and, after several years of use, of breast cancer and endometrial cancer – although this last risk is reduced if the HRT contains a progestogen. You and your doctor can work together to determine whether HRT is right for you and how long you can remain on it.

Women without a uterus (following hysterectomy) may take oestrogen replacement therapy on its own without a progestogen. When oestrogen is used alone, the treatment is called *unopposed oestrogen therapy* because progestogen isn't included to oppose the effects of oestrogen.

Between the 1950s and 1970s, doctors routinely prescribed *oestrogen* on its own to treat menopausal symptoms in all women, including women with a uterus. As the incidence of endometrial cancer in menopausal women climbed during this period, researchers realised that taking oestrogen therapy alone increases the risk of menopausal women developing endometrial cancer. Researchers also discovered that adding in a progestogen (a synthetic version of *progesterone*) for a few days each month lowers the risk of endometrial cancer.

Oestrogen stimulates growth of the *endometrium* (uterine lining) to make a nice soft nest for a fertilised egg. Part of this stimulation involves encouraging the overgrowth of endometrial cells. If this stimulation continues unchecked, the womb lining cells and glands enlarge – a medical condition known as *cystic hyperplasia*. Left untreated, this eventually leads to abnormal cell changes that can trigger endometrial cancer. Progestogen opposes this action of oestrogen and acts on the womb lining so that the womb cells and glands stop proliferating and start to mature. This protects against the development of cystic hyperplasia.

Women who no longer have a womb due to hysterectomy are the only women who should receive oestrogen alone. Without a uterus, their chances of developing uterine cancer drop to zero. (Take a look at the 'Unopposed oestrogen therapy' section later in this chapter for more info.) For most other women, a combination of oestrogen and progestogen is necessary.

Slaying the symptoms

Some women's perimenopausal symptoms are so severe that they interfere with their family life, career, self-esteem, or happiness.

Taking hormone replacement therapy to alleviate the symptoms of perimenopause, such as hot flushes, vaginal dryness, disrupted sleep, mood swings, memory changes, and so on, works fabulously for many women. (Check out the Cheat Sheet and Chapter 3 for a full rundown of perimenopausal and menopausal symptoms.) Despite studies showing the health risks associated with HRT, many women wouldn't want to go without HRT because their perimenopausal symptoms threaten their enjoyment of life.

Other women prefer to use complementary therapies to alleviate the symptoms associated with perimenopause, however, and you can check out these in Chapter 16.

Preventing serious health problems with HRT

In 1900, you could expect to live to a ripe old age of 50 – barely into menopause. Thanks to improvements in nutrition and healthcare, the average lifespan is now nearly 80 years – way beyond menopause. If you're an average woman (or better than average), you should definitely consider shifting to a healthier lifestyle. You may also want to consider hormone replacement therapy. Here's why:

Oestrogen keeps the engine that is your body running smoothly, and you're going to drive this engine for quite some time (unlike women in historical times who only drove their engine while new). Think about how you maintain your body. It's one thing to have a low oil level when you're just on a short trip, but taking a long-distance journey when you're low on oil is a completely different story. Your engine will burn up long before you reach the end of your road. Just like you routinely check your car and top up its oil level when necessary (hopefully before noticing a problem), you need to intervene with a healthy diet, lifestyle, and sometimes medicine – even when you're not sick – to help keep your body's engine running smoothly.

Some of the health problems standing in the way of staying active and comfortable are related to the fact that women produce lower levels of oestrogen after the menopause – a period that may last for 30 or more years. Low levels of oestrogen can lead to health issues such as

- ✔ Coronary heart disease (angina and heart attack)
- ✔ Hardening of the arteries
- ✔ High blood pressure
- ✔ Increased risk of certain cancers
- ✔ Osteoporosis

Although HRT has beneficial effects on your bones, your main defence against these problems is a healthy diet, lifestyle, and preventive medicine. (See Part IV: Lifestyle Issues for Menopause and Beyond for lots of suggestions in these areas.)

Think of hormone replacement therapy as representing one leg of a four-legged stool. HRT provides greater benefit to women who also eat a healthy diet, get regular exercise, and visit their doctor regularly. You can explore the benefits and risks of HRT and the ramifications of long-term use in greater detail in Chapter 15.

Ticking through the Treatments

Every woman's body is different, and you can choose from a variety of regimens and many different types of HRT to suit your own circumstances. In this section we aim to help you understand the different types of treatment available, and why they are used.

Unopposed oestrogen therapy

Unopposed oestrogen therapy refers to a treatment programme in which you receive only oestrogen without a progestogen (a synthetic form of progesterone).

Doctors use unopposed oestrogen-only HRT if you have no uterus (due to a hysterectomy), because taking oestrogen without progestogen can lead to endometrial cancer.

If you have a history of blood-clotting problems such as deep-vein thrombosis, your doctor must weigh the benefits versus the risks of HRT for you. In general, blood-clotting problems are associated with high dosages of oestrogen – particularly in smokers. Regardless of whether you smoke, your doctor will probably start you on the lowest dosage of HRT available and move you to a higher dose only if the lowest dose doesn't relieve your symptoms. Low-dosage oestrogen reduces your risk of blood clotting.

Some evidence shows that the oestradiol form of oestrogen is less likely to contribute to clotting problems than the conjugated types of oestrogen. Oestrogen patches, gels, and nasal sprays don't send oestrogen straight to your liver, and so these forms of oestrogen are the delivery method of choice to avoid clotting problems. Oral tablets, on the other hand, after absorption in your intestines, go straight to your liver before circulating around your body. As the liver breaks down hormones, much larger doses are needed with oral medications compared with doses absorbed through the skin.

If you have a liver or gall bladder disease or high blood pressure, discuss these conditions with your doctor before using any type of oestrogen.

Treatment methods

First, your doctor evaluates your symptoms and hormone levels to establish an appropriate dosage – usually, the minimum effective dose is used for the shortest duration of time. You may take an oestrogen pill every day or use a patch that you apply to your abdomen once or twice a week – the timing depends on the brand and your doctor's recommendations. An oestrogen gel that you apply to your skin daily is also available, as is an oestrogen nasal spray, which you use once a day.

Benefits

Taking unopposed oestrogen boosts the amount of oestrogen circulating in your bloodstream. This boost alleviates a variety of symptoms including:

- **Headaches:** Oestrogen increases blood flow by relaxing blood vessels.

- **Hot flushes, heart palpitations, and anxiety:** Oestrogen lowers your production of adrenaline, the stress hormone that makes your heart race and your blood vessels dilate.

✔ **Interrupted sleep:** Oestrogen alleviates hot flushes and increases sero-tonin production, helping you sleep through the night.

✔ **Memory lapses:** Oestrogen promotes communication among nerve cells in the brain.

✔ **Mood swings and irritability:** Oestrogen increases serotonin production to produce an antidepressant action.

✔ **Vaginal dryness and atrophy, frequent urination, and urinary inconti-nence:** Oestrogen helps to moisturise your urogenital tissues, keeping them pliable enough to avoid these problems.

Oestrogen on its own also has beneficial effects on bone maintenance, cho-lesterol levels, clotting factors, and the health of your blood vessels and heart tissue. (Check out Chapter 2 for more information on oestrogen.)

Taking unopposed oestrogen can also eliminate the premenstrual-syndrome-like side effects of bloating, breast tenderness, and similar symptoms that can occur due to the effects of natural progesterone in your body.

Side effects

Side effects of oestrogen replacement include nausea, breast fullness or ten-derness, headache, dizziness, leg cramps, vaginal candida, an increase in *triglycerides* (a type of fat in your blood), and an increase in blood pressure. These side effects are often reduced or eliminated if your doctor decreases your dosage or switches you from the pill form of oestrogen to an *oestradiol* (active oestrogen) patch or gel that you apply to your skin, as sometimes side effects reflect a reaction to a dye or other inactive 'filler' ingredient in an oestrogen tablet. These side effects may include joint aches, muscle aches, skin irritation, and a burning sensation when urinating.

Cautions

Unopposed oestrogen therapy is *not* suitable for any woman who still has a uterus because of the risk of endometrial cancer. Other reasons not to use this type of HRT include a history of breast cancer or other oestrogen-dependent cancer (such as vaginal cancer), undiagnosed vaginal bleeding, active blood clotting problems such as deep-vein thrombosis or recent heart attack, and abnormal liver function. Your doctor should ensure that you are eligible for treatment before prescribing any kind of HRT for you.

If you have had a hysterectomy and but have a family history of breast cancer, the answer isn't so clear. Have a frank discussion with your doctor to decide whether this type of therapy is right for you.

Stay away from oestrogen therapy if you're pregnant or breastfeeding!

Combined oestrogen and progestogen therapy

Combination therapy means taking a combination of oestrogen plus a progestogen (the synthetic form of progesterone) rather than taking only oestrogen. The progestogen is usually given in the tablet, in the patch, or is delivered continually into your womb via a special type of coil known as the intra-uterine system (IUS). A synthetic hormone called tibolone is also available, which provides both oestrogen and progestogen activity in a single preparation.

Combining oestrogen with a progestogen provides the benefits of oestrogen while reducing the risk of endometrial cancer that taking unopposed oestrogen can heighten. The down side is that progestogen slightly reduces some of the benefits of oestrogen. The sole purpose of including progestogen in hormone replacement therapy is to reduce your risk of endometrial cancer, which may otherwise be raised by taking oestrogen. If you have not had your uterus removed and you elect to take hormone replacement therapy, a doctor always puts you on a form of combination HRT.

Treatment methods

Combination hormone replacement therapy comes in two basic forms: Cyclic and continuous combination therapy. And cyclical combination therapy also has a few different options for you to choose from. The form you use depends on your individual circumstances and symptoms.

- ✔ **Cyclic combination therapy:** With this form, you take oestrogen and progestogen in a cycle. Generally the first part of the cycle involves oestrogen, and the second part involves oestrogen plus progestogen. This combination triggers a period because the progestogen tells your uterus to shed its endometrial lining.

  'But I thought menopause meant that you don't have a period,' you say? Well you're right. You're not technically having a menstrual period; you're having a vaginal hormone-withdrawal bleed. Drugs, not ovulation, trigger the periods that come with hormone replacement therapy. Cyclic hormone replacement therapy gives most women a predictable pattern of vaginal bleeding, which continues for as long as the HRT is prescribed.

  Your doctor may recommend one of two common cyclic combination programmes, as follows:

  - In one regimen, you take oestrogen every day of the month and progestogen is added in for the last 10 to 14 days of each cycle.

  - In the other cyclic combination regimen, you take oestrogen alone for 11 days, then oestrogen and progestogen together for 10 days. Then you have a seven-day interval with no medication. You can expect to bleed when you're not taking the medication. Some people refer to this regimen as *sequential combination therapy* because you take the oestrogen and progestogen in a sequence.

✔ **Continuous combined (or continuous opposed) therapy:** With this form of HRT, you take oestrogen and progestogen together every day. This approach seems to provide the following benefits:

- Lower risk of endometrial cancer

- Cessation of periods after six months or a year

- Fewer progestogen-related side effects in some women (see the following 'Side effects' section), especially bleeding

Pills and patches on the market today combine the two hormones making them easy to use. If you're bothered by side effects, talk with your doctor about experimenting with different dosages or forms to make you more comfortable.

Some women on combination therapy don't like the side effects they feel on the days they take the progestogen. Never stop taking the progestogen without consulting your doctor, and always take the progestogen for the exact length of time prescribed. Taking just oestrogen can lead to endometrial cancer. (For more information, see 'Unopposed oestrogen therapy' earlier in this chapter.)

Certain progestogens are derived from testosterone and can help women who complain of low libido (sex drive) during and after menopause. The generic name for this progestogen is *norethisterone*. Although norethisterone reduces many of the progestogen side effects, doctors do not recommend it for women with high LDL-cholesterol or triglyceride levels. Some doctors may prescribe testosterone for postmenopausal women with low sex drive in the form of a gel or implant, but doing so is controversial in the UK.

Benefits

Combination therapy gives you the benefits of oestrogen without the increased risks of endometrial cancer that taking oestrogen alone entails.

Continuous hormone replacement therapy causes fewer side effects in women who are several years beyond menopause than in younger women. Continuous hormone replacement therapy causes fewer premenstrual-like symptoms than cyclic hormone replacement therapy. If you are tired of tampons, you may like to know that a third of women stop bleeding when they start continuous combination therapy, many women stop monthly bleeding after two to three months, and most women stop monthly bleeding after one year of therapy. But proper dosages and delivery forms are needed to curb the side effects of progestogen, which may occur if you take too high a dose continuously.

If you require contraception, another option is to use the intra-uterine system (IUS), which is basically a contraceptive device that releases a small amount of progestogen directly into the womb. This progestogen protects against overgrowth of the womb lining. If you are fitted with an IUS, you can use oestrogen-only HRT just as if you did not have a uterus. The IUS is especially helpful for women with heavy periods as, after one year, many women using the IUS have few if any periods. When used to oppose oestrogen replacement, the IUS is effective for four years before needing replacement. As the dose of progestogen is very low, and little is absorbed into the circulation, the IUS has few, if any, progestogen-related side effects.

Side effects

Some women have a hard enough time tolerating their own progesterone. Tolerating its synthetic cousin, progestogen, is no easier. Progesterone and progestogen can cause many premenstrual-syndrome-like symptoms, including

- Acne
- Bloating
- Depression
- Weight gain

Cautions

Women with a history of breast cancer should not take hormone replacement therapy, and those with a family history of breast cancer should consider the risks carefully. Although initially it was thought that HRT reduced the risk of coronary heart disease this is no longer certain. Women shouldn't take hormone replacement therapy to prevent coronary heart disease or to reduce the risk of heart attack, according to the recent results of the Women's Health Initiative study (see Chapter 11).

Women who have heart disease, uncontrolled diabetes, high blood pressure, high triglyceride levels, fibromyalgia, or depression aren't good candidates for continuous combination therapy, because taking progestogen every day often exacerbates these conditions.

Selective Oestrogen Receptor Modulators

Meet the stealth bombers of the hormone replacement therapy world – selective oestrogen receptor modulators. Oddly for us, these are often referred to as SERMs, not SORMs, as oestrogen is spelled with an e – estrogen – in the US, where brainy boffins invented these drugs.

SERMs are super-duper designer drugs that target specific types of oestrogen receptors (those areas that welcome and use oestrogen) while blocking oestrogen receptors in other parts of the body. SERMs don't contain oestrogen. They stimulate oestrogen receptors in the bone, brain, and cardiovascular system, but block the receptors in the breast and uterus.

SERMs provide the benefits of oestrogen to specific parts of the body without the drawbacks – and of course, the biggest drawback is the increased risk of breast cancer. At present, two SERMs are available in the UK, but others are in the pipeline:

- **Raloxifene:** Used for the treatment and prevention of postmenopausal osteoporosis. Raloxifene builds new bone and slows down the destruction of old bone during the bone maintenance process. Raloxifene, like tamoxifen, seems to provide an improvement in blood cholesterol, lowering bad cholesterol and total cholesterol slightly. This SERM doesn't increase your risk of endometrial or breast cancer.

- **Tamoxifen:** Designed for women with specific types of breast cancer, to prevent further recurrence. Tamoxifen is generally used in conjunction with other forms of treatment, such as surgery or chemotherapy. Research shows that tamoxifen provides benefits similar to hormone replacement therapy, including lowering blood cholesterol and improving bone density.

Treatment methods

Both tamoxifen and raloxifene are available in pill form and are taken according to your doctor's instructions.

Benefits

SERMs may reduce bone loss in menopausal women, but not as well as oestrogen does. SERMs reduce the risk of breast cancer in women if taken for no more than five years. Unlike combination hormone replacement therapy, SERMs have no negative effects on blood lipids, so they won't raise your triglyceride or LDL-cholesterol levels.

Research into SERMs is ongoing, and new types of SERM are on their way. Targeting specific oestrogen receptors to stimulate is a promising way to help women stay comfortable and healthy during and after menopause.

Side effects

Unfortunately, SERMs do have a few side effects, including the following:

- Hot flushes
- Insomnia
- Slightly increased risk of endometrial cancer (with tamoxifen)

SERMs are beneficial to your blood cholesterol, but they do increase the risk of blood clots in your veins and lungs and may lead to strokes.

Cautions

If you are at risk of cardiovascular problems, you should avoid SERMs. Women with hot flushes don't tolerate SERMs well because these drugs tend to make symptoms worse.

Pondering Pills, Patches, and Pomades: A Smorgasbord of Delivery Options

Over the years, scientists have worked hard to provide hormone replacement therapy that maximises the benefits and minimises the side effects and inconveniences. The result of all this effort is a buffet of choices. Basically, you have five paths to choose from to deliver hormone replacement therapy to your bloodstream:

- ✔ Your mouth (pill)
- ✔ Your skin (patches or gel)
- ✔ Your vagina (cream, gel, or ring)
- ✔ Your nose (nasal spray)
- ✔ Under your skin (implant)

The various delivery systems offer choices to suit the personal and physiological preferences of a diverse group of women. You and your doctor can experiment to find the delivery methods and dosages most effective for you.

In the following sections, we describe the various delivery systems and the benefits and drawbacks of each. We also go through the different types of hormones used in hormone replacement therapy.

Popping pills

Swallowing a pill or tablet is a traditional way of ingesting medication, so understanding and performing the procedure correctly is easy. Getting the exact dose that your doctor orders is also simple because the prescribed dosage is already loaded in the pill and you read the frequency on the label.

By the time you reach the age of 60 or 70, however, you may take various medications. For example, many women take a multivitamin, extra calcium, blood-pressure medication, maybe something to reduce indigestion, and so on and so on. An additional pill in the parade may be a pain.

Pasting on a patch

Patches deliver drugs through your skin. Two or three years ago, bulky patches with a skin-irritating reservoir of alcohol delivered the hormone. Today's patches are known as *matrix patches* because the hormone is actually incorporated into the adhesive that sticks it to your skin. These patches are much smaller, thinner, and less likely to irritate your skin than the patches of days gone by.

Patches have some advantages over other forms of HRT delivery:

- ✔ You put them on just once or twice a week.
- ✔ They deliver a constant supply of hormone so that you have more consistent hormone levels in your blood.
- ✔ They're easier on your liver and digestive tract than pills as they bypass these parts of your body and go straight into your bloodstream.

The only real problem you may have with a patch is that it may irritate your skin. This problem is, however, unusual.

Slathering on a gel

You can apply oestrogen in the form of a gel, rather like applying body lotion. Once a day, you squirt out one to four measures of the gel from its handy pump and apply the gel over an area of your skin, such as your lower trunk, inner thighs, arms, or shoulders. The size of the area to cover is usually around twice the size of your hand. Do not apply the gel near your breasts, face, or vulva. You need to wait five minutes or so for the gel to dry before putting on clothes, and then wait at least an hour before washing the treated area – otherwise you wash it off before it can be absorbed.

Don't touch other people with the treated area of skin – especially your male partner – so don't apply it just before sex! Otherwise someone else may absorb your hormones – not a good idea.

Many women find oestrogen gel the bee's knees, because of the ease with which it can be applied. If you still have your womb, you can use oestrogen gel provided that you take cyclical progestogen for 12 days of each cycle or have the intra-uterine system fitted.

Applying vaginal creams

Your vaginal lining responds quickly to treatments applied directly to the area. Some women like vaginal creams because they deliver the hormones localised in a small area.

If you're treating vaginal dryness or atrophy but you worry about breast and endometrial cancer, vaginal cream may be a good choice. For example, an oestrogen cream relieves vaginal dryness and atrophy but doesn't increase your risk of breast cancer because the dosage is low and the oestrogen stays put.

Creams are effective for treating your vagina, but they do nothing for your hot flushes, mood swings, bones, or blood cholesterol.

Cream applicators are often cumbersome to load and can make the whole process difficult and inexact. You may get more or less of a dose than you expected, and inevitably you lose cream from the vagina after the application. So you're never really sure exactly how much cream you've truly applied and how much you've lost. You may feel like putting a bit more in the applicator to compensate, but you don't know how much extra to add. Because applying creams is cumbersome, some women just quit using the cream or don't apply the cream on a proper schedule.

Vaginal oestrogen tablets are also available. These tablets are easy to apply into the vagina (*don't swallow them!*), give a precise dose, and make less of a mess than vaginal creams. One of these tablets is about the size of a baby aspirin. You insert the tablet high into your vagina with an applicator like you'd use for a tampon, only narrower. The pill dissolves slowly inside your body and releases small amounts of oestrogen. You administer these pills about twice a week.

Slipping on a ring

The ring we refer to here doesn't go on your finger: You place it in your vagina. Your doctor usually inserts the flexible, hormone-containing ring initially. The ring stays in place continuously until changed – usually every

90 days. The ring slowly delivers an even supply of hormones into your bloodstream. The dosage is very low, so it doesn't stimulate growth of your endometrial lining.

Don't worry: The ring is out of the way. If you've used a diaphragm, the ring isn't that much different (although, of course, the ring is not a contraceptive). Some women have a problem tolerating the ring because they have a short or narrow vagina. You can pop out the ring before using the bathroom (so that it doesn't ping out into the toilet) and before sex if your partner feels the ring and finds it off-putting – just remember to put it back in afterwards.

A vaginal ring is a great option if you have vaginal and urinary tract symptoms. However, the ring doesn't provide all the other health benefits of oestrogen such as relief of perimenopausal symptoms and improved bone maintenance.

Squirting a nasal spray

If you don't mind squirting oestrogen up your nose, then a nasal spray may be an option for you. You spray once a day into each nostril, every day, or for 21–28 days with a 2–7 day treatment-free interval. If one dose per nostril isn't enough to control your symptoms, you can increase up to four sprays a day in divided doses. If you still have your womb, you use the spray with cyclical progestogen for at least 12 days per cycle. If your nose is runny, blow first and then spray. If you have a bad cold and a blocked up nose, you can spray into your mouth between your cheek and gum, but you have to double your normal dose if you choose this option.

The most frequently reported side effects of the oestrogen nasal spray are prickling or tingling sensations inside the nose, sneezing, and runny nose, and these effects are usually mild. Whatever you do, don't confuse the nasal spray with the other sprays in your bathroom cabinet such as hairspray, mouth freshener or perfume!

Investigating implants

If you find it difficult to remember to take a tablet or apply a patch, spray or gel, then perhaps an implant may suit you best. These are most suitable for women who have had a hysterectomy and removal of both ovaries. Implants are often inserted during the operation to prevent a sudden onset of severe surgical menopausal symptoms. If you have an implant inserted after a hysterectomy, your doctor first numbs the insertion site with local anaesthetic and then inserts a hollow needle (called a *trocar*) into the fat under your skin. The doctor pushes an oestrogen pellet out of the end of the needle and into the fat. If you no longer have ovaries, some doctors prefer to insert both oestrogen and testosterone pellets to help to maintain your sex drive. If you still have a uterus, you can have an oestrogen implant if your doctor thinks that having one is the best option for you, but you need cyclical progestogen or an intra-uterine system to protect your womb lining from cystic hyperplasia, (which we explain in 'Defining Hormone Replacement Therapy' earlier in this chapter). Implants are reinserted as required, usually every 4–8 months. Your doctor may check your blood oestrogen levels to tell when you need your next implant.

Searching for Sources

Are you the type of person who eats only organic foods? Do you opt for fresh veggies over the canned variety? Do you grab bottled water because of that weird smell in your water at home? If you answered yes to any of these questions, you may wonder how to maintain this level of purity in your hormones too.

Unfortunately, deciding what's 'natural' when it comes to hormone replacement therapy is difficult. Like beauty, natural HRT is in the eye of the beholder. You can look at 'natural' in a couple of ways:

- ✔ 'Natural' can mean similar to what you already have in your body. In the laboratory, scientists can replicate the exact molecular structure of human hormones. The results are identical to human hormones but without the stray bits that exist in all animal hormones. So these hormones have the same structure as natural human hormones, but they're made in a lab, so they're synthetic but nature-identical.

- ✔ 'Natural' can also mean coming from nature – plants and animals. Some hormones are derived from plants but are modified to produce a beneficial effect in our bodies. Other hormones come from animals. So, these natural hormones come from nature, but they're not *natural* to humans.

So, 'natural' isn't really a good term for describing the hormones used for hormone replacement therapy. The next section gives you the source of the hormones – you decide whether you consider it natural or not.

Oestrogen

Scientists have found a variety of sources from which to make oestrogen. But before you get started with the recipes for HRT, a quick reminder about the ins and outs of oestrogen is in order. Three types of oestrogen exist: oestradiol, oestrone, and oestriol – for the whole story, refer to Chapter 2:

- ✔ **Oestradiol** is the biologically active type of oestrogen and the most potent form of human oestrogen. Oestradiol's a player in hundreds of bodily functions.

- ✔ **Oestrone** isn't the workhorse that oestradiol is. Oestrone is more like the warehouse variety of oestrogen that's stored in your body fat. It is turned into oestradiol, but only in premenopausal ovaries.

- ✔ **Oestriol** – forget about it (in this context anyway). Oestriol is mostly found in pregnant women.

Now that that's taken care of, here are the sources of oestrogen that scientists have come up with:

- ✔ **Conjugated equine oestrogen:** Made from the urine of pregnant horses. Some of the most-prescribed oestrogens used in hormone replacement therapy are conjugated equine oestrogens. This type of oestrogen has the least amount of oestradiol, but it delivers lots of oestrone and a significant amount of *equilin,* an oestrogen found in horses. Although equilins are great for female horses, doctors occupy both sides of the fence on the subject of whether equilin is beneficial to human females. Conjugated equine oestrogen is available in pill and cream form.

- ✔ **Oestradiol oestrogen:** Derived from soybeans and/or wild yams. These oestrogens are chemically identical to human oestradiol oestrogen. Oestradiol oestrogen is available in every delivery method – pill, cream, ring, gel, spray, patch and implant. (Check out 'Pondering Pills, Patches, and Pomades: A Smorgasbord of Delivery Options' earlier in this chapter for more info.) In fact, oestradiol's the only type of oestrogen used in the patch.

- ✔ **Esterified oestrogen:** Made from soybeans and/or wild yams (sometimes referred to as Mexican yams). Esterified oestrogen provides high levels of oestrone and much lower levels of oestradiol oestrogen, but it can help maintain bone and improve perimenopausal symptoms and lipid profiles in the blood. Esterified oestrogen is available as a pill.

- ✔ **Estropipate:** Also known as *piperazine oestrogen sulphate.* Available as a pill or cream, this synthetic form of oestrogen is chemically similar, but not identical, to human oestrone. A drawback of estropipate is that it may aggravate pain in women who have muscle- or bladder-pain syndromes.

✔ **Micronised oestradiol:** Provides the same type of active oestrogen (oestradiol) that the ovaries produce naturally. The oestradiol is produced synthetically (in the lab) from soybeans.

Micronisation means that the particles are small enough to enter your bloodstream before your digestive system destroys them. So here we go with the 'What's natural and what's not?' discussion. Micronised oestradiol is made from a 'natural' plant, but technicians tweak it in the lab so that your body can use it. You take this oestradiol as a pill.

Some doctors claim that using a form of oestrogen that's molecularly similar to human oestradiol is no more beneficial to women than oestrogen products derived from pregnant mares; others claim that it makes a world of difference.

Progestogen

Most of the side effects attributed to hormone replacement therapy are the result of the progestogen, but progestogen protects you from developing endometrial cancer. Because every woman's body is different, you and your doctor may need to experiment to figure out which progestogen is right for you.

Adding progestogen to the hormone replacement therapy mix does seem to reduce the benefits oestrogen can have on your cholesterol levels and increase changes to your mood.

Companies market three types of progestogen:

✔ **Progesterone:** Even though this is identical to the human hormone produced by the ovary in premenopausal women. Progesterone is available as a vaginal gel or pessaries (and as an injection to treat heavy menstrual bleeding).

✔ **Progestogens derived from progesterone:** Includes medroxyprogesterone acetate (MPA) and dydrogesterone. These are used to oppose oestrogen HRT during the last half of each oestrogen HRT cycle. They are available as tablets.

✔ **Progestogens derived from testosterone:** Includes norethisterone and norgestrel. Newer progestogens are derived from norgestrel, and include desogestrel, norgestimate, and gestodene. Levonorgestrel is the active form of norgestrel and has twice its activity. These progestogens have fewer side effects than MPA and provide a libido boost in some women. These progestogens aren't recommended for women with high cholesterol or low HDL (the 'good' cholesterol) levels. They are available in various pills and patches.

Combinations of oestrogen and progestogen

For convenience, you may want to take oestrogen and progestogen as a combination in a single pill or patch. Many brands of HRT tablet provide sequential combinations of oestrogen and progestogen: You start off taking oestrogen-only at the beginning of the month, and then take a different-coloured tablet containing both oestrogen and progestogen during the second half of the month. Some brands contain three different-coloured pills in a calendar pack, so you start by taking a higher dose of oestrogen, then oestrogen plus progestogen, and then a lower dose of oestrogen for the remainder of the month.

Some packs combine an oestrogen patch with progestogen tablets, so that you use just the patch at the beginning of your cycle, and then the patch plus the tablet during the second half of the cycle. The more popular option is to use patches that allow both oestrogen and the progestogen to absorb through your skin at the same time. This way, you don't need to remember the tablet.

With some brands you use the combination patch continuously, changing it as often as advised. With other brands you use an oestrogen-only patch for two weeks, followed with a combined oestrogen and progestogen patch for two weeks.

Tibolone is an unusual synthetic hormone that provides oestrogen, progestogen, and weak testosterone activity from one source. Neither tibolone nor continuous combined preparations of HRT are suitable for use during perimenopause or within 12 months of your last menstrual period as they can trigger irregular bleeding.

As combination HRT regimes vary so much, always follow your doctor's advice and read the instructions inside each pack.

TECHNICAL STUFF

Targeting your hormone levels after menopause

So just how much active oestrogen do you need pulsing through your body to keep you healthy and comfortable?

Most experts in the field agree that, after menopause, you don't need oestrogen levels as high as in your premenopausal years.

The normal range of plasma oestradiol during the menstrual cycle of premenopausal women is between 200 and 1200 pmol/L (that's picomols per litre). After menopause, oestradiol levels without hormone replacement are usually less than 100 pmol/L.

Research suggests that a plasma oestradiol level of at least 300 pmol/L is necessary to improve your bone density. An implant containing 25mg oestradiol gives an average oestradiol level of around 320 pmol/L, and most women obtain good energy, mood, sleep, and memory levels when blood levels of oestradiol are at this level or above, although some women need a higher dose.

Oestradiol levels that are persistently below 300 pmol/L typically result in hot flushes, interrupted sleep, mood swings, and other annoying menopausal symptoms. Your risk of bone loss and cardiovascular issues also increases. So, your doctor's target is to get your oestradiol levels between 300 pmol/L and 500 pmol/L. Some studies have found that higher oestradiol levels are associated with the development of psychological symptoms that resemble those of dependency.

Doing the Dosing

The guideline that every doctor follows is: Use the smallest effective dose for the shortest amount of time, to alleviate symptoms while reducing the health risks. That said, women react to hormone supplements differently. No one knows why a particular regimen causes one woman to experience side effects and another to sing its praises from the rooftop.

Your doctor reviews your personal medical history, your family medical history, and the results of your physical examination and tests. Share your personal preferences and prejudices with your doctor at this time as well. For example, do you have a hard time swallowing pills? Do you forget to take medicine? Are you determined to throw away the tampons as soon as possible?

If you have issues with your libido, ask your doctor to take your libido into account when prescribing hormone replacement therapy. Convenience is also an issue: For example, how many other medications you take (do you really want to take more pills or use a patch?), the cost, and how anxious you are to stop bleeding every month. As far as the latter issue goes, *sequential/ cyclical therapy* (taking oestrogen for part of the month and progestogen another part of the month) results in continuing your periods for some time, but *continuous combination therapy* (taking both oestrogen and progestogen at the same time every day) generally stops your periods. SERMs, (which we describe above in 'Selective Oestrogen Receptor Modulators') also eliminate your periods.

Continuous combined HRT (including tibolone) is not suitable for use in the perimenopause or within 12 months of your last menstrual period, as it can cause irregular bleeding.

Your doctor may need to experiment with these different products to find the right one for you – that is, a product that eliminates your symptoms while causing the fewest side effects.

Most doctors start out using standard low doses and increase the dose slowly if necessary. With hormone replacement therapy, one size doesn't fit all. If you are using an oestradiol implant, your doctor may take a blood sample to figure out where your hormones are and to work out when best to insert your next implant so that your hormones are in the appropriate target range (see the sidebar 'Targeting your hormone levels after menopause' in this chapter).

Chapter 11

Focusing on HRT and Your Heart

. . . .

In This Chapter

▶ Recognising the effects of each hormone on your heart's health

▶ Brushing up on how hormones keep your cardiovascular system healthy

▶ Discovering the latest research on hormone replacement therapy, your blood vessels, and your heart

. . . .

*U*ntil the results of the Women's Health Initiative (WHI) study were released in 2002, most medics thought that hormone replacement therapy (HRT) was beneficial for your heart. Although your body's own oestrogen definitely lowers your risk of heart disease and keeps your blood cholesterol healthy *during your reproductive years,* HRT is probably not the godsend for menopausal women that most experts originally thought.

The research into whether HRT actually makes for a healthier cardiovascular system is all over the place. Researchers are still studying this issue after decades, but some of the trials are small or biased in their selection of people to study. So doctors and medical groups have all been drawing their own conclusions as to which study to believe – if you ask 50 different doctors for their medical opinion on this topic, you are likely to get 50 different answers.

You need to seriously consider cardiovascular issues because, whether you're talking about stroke, high blood pressure, or heart attack, more women than men die from cardiovascular disease.

This chapter helps you to understand the 'whats' and 'hows' behind the beneficial effects that hormone replacement therapy has on your cardiovascular system and fills you in on the drawbacks. It also covers the findings of the WHI study in each area that it examines. With this information in hand, you can make better long-term decisions about how to live a healthy life during perimenopause and menopause and how to cope with the cardiovascular risks that increase with age. (But, before you make any decisions, check out the other chapters on HRT (and the alternatives) in this book – Chapter 10 and Chapters 12–17.)

Meeting the Players: Hormones and Your Heart

As far as your sex hormones go, oestrogen, progesterone, and testosterone play different roles in your cardiovascular system, so you probably want to know what they do for a living. In the following sections we outline what these hormones do for your blood, blood vessels, and heart before the menopause. The trick to hormone replacement therapy is finding the right level and balance of hormones that protects your heart without raising your risks of heart attack, stroke, abnormal blood clots, and breast cancer.

The star: Oestrogen

Because oestrogen protects your cardiovascular system, women have around ten-years as a grace period before the risk of developing heart disease increases, in comparison with men. Most of the cardiovascular benefits attributed to hormone replacement therapy are due to the protective nature of oestrogen.

Take a look at how oestrogen works on your cardiovascular system:

- ✔ Oestrogen decreases blood pressure when given via a skin patch.
- ✔ Oestrogen decreases triglycerides.
- ✔ Oestrogen improves blood flow in your coronary arteries.
- ✔ Oestrogen increases 'good' HDL cholesterol levels.
- ✔ Oestrogen reduces fibrinogen, which may then lower your risk of blood clots.
- ✔ Oestrogen reduces the build up of plaque in your coronary arteries.
- ✔ Oestrogen relaxes artery walls to help dilate blood vessels and avoid spasms.

But oestrogen replacement can also have the following negative effects:

- ✔ Increases blood clots (deep-vein thrombosis) at high levels
- ✔ Increases triglycerides when taken as a pill
- ✔ A skin-patch doesn't effect HDL and LDL levels for six months

Paying attention to the type of oestrogen you take, and the delivery mechanism you use can help to avoid these problems. As you can see from the list above, different methods of delivery can produce different results. (For more details on the advantages and disadvantages of different oestrogen-delivery forms, refer to Chapter 10.)

Continuously reviewing your HRT regimen throughout your life is important. Your health conditions can change, which may mean that you need to change your programme.

The supporting actor: Progesterone

Progesterone's main function is to prepare your body for pregnancy. When progesterone levels peak, most women feel bloated and ravenously hungry. Your breasts may feel tender and enlarged. If your egg isn't fertilised, progesterone levels drop, you have your period, and these symptoms go away.

So why in the world would anyone knowingly ask women to take this hormone after they finally rid their systems of it? Researchers and doctors haven't always understood the benefits of progesterone on normal body functioning. But medical experts now know that oestrogen, when taken alone, can increase your risk of endometrial (uterine) cancer. So, doctors add a *progestogen* – synthetic progesterone – to nearly all HRT programmes to lower your risk of endometrial cancer. The discovery that progestogen can limit the cancer risk that comes with oestrogen-only therapy is a huge benefit for menopausal women. (Women who have had their uterus surgically removed don't receive progestogen because they no longer have to worry about uterine cancer.)

Although progestogen reduces your risk of endometrial cancer, it has negative effects on your cardiovascular system. In particular, progestogen:

- ✔ Increases triglycerides (very low-density lipids – nearly all fat)
- ✔ Lowers HDL ('good' cholesterol) levels
- ✔ Lowers your sensitivity to insulin, which affects your ability to process glucose (this effect is of great concern to people with diabetes)
- ✔ Tends to make you store fats instead of breaking them down

With the variety of progestogens on the market today, some of these problems are minimal. Your doctor can scrutinise your regimen to make sure that you get the proper dosage, the proper delivery form, and the proper type of progestogen. For more information on the advantages and disadvantages of various hormone regimens, refer to Chapter 10.

Your doctor must perform an individual assessment of you and your needs to determine the right HRT regimen for you.

The assistant: Testosterone

Women's bodies naturally produce testosterone, a so-called male hormone, although at much lower levels than are found in men (just as well if you don't fancy sporting a six-pack and moustache). When given with *oestradiol* (the active form of oestrogen), testosterone helps to relax and dilate your blood vessels, improving the flow of blood. If you take testosterone on its own with no oestradiol, it seems to have the opposite effect, promoting plaque build-up on vessel walls. Although some doctors prescribe testosterone to menopausal women, this is still controversial in the UK.

Testosterone treatment is a touchy subject, so work with your doctor to make sure that your hormone replacement therapy promotes a healthy balance in your hormone levels. When women take testosterone along with oestrogen, some of the negative effects of testosterone are reversed according to newer studies. If testosterone is part of your HRT regimen, check that your doctor religiously monitors your blood cholesterol balance and modifies treatment as needed.

Understanding the Significance of the Women's Health Initiative Study

The *Women's Health Initiative* (WHI) study, which stirred the HRT debate early in 2002, is much better designed than previous studies. Its results are based on 16,000 participants and solid research methods. The study has one problem, however: The WHI studied only one type of hormone replacement therapy – conjugated equine oestrogen combined with MPA (medroxyprogesterone acetate) progestogen. Although doctors commonly prescribe this type of hormone replacement therapy in the United States, it is less common in the UK, and the exact doses used (0.625mg conjugated equine oestrogen plus 2.5mg MPA) are not available on prescription in the UK.

The results of the WHI study are important, as they scientifically document the effects of this particular course of therapy on women's health. We think that these new results are important, and so we provide you with their conclusions throughout this chapter. But we also provide you with information on the use of unopposed oestrogen and research from other studies evaluating the use of oestrogen and progesterone. Unfortunately, the WHI study does not answer all the questions concerning hormone replacement therapy and heart disease.

Skimming the Fat: HRT and Your Blood

Coronary heart disease is due to hardening and furring up of the coronary arteries that supply blood, oxygen, and nutrients to your heart muscle. Over the years, fat is deposited on the walls of your blood vessels and attracts other substances that eventually get capped with a calcium layer, to form *plaque*. This process, called *atherosclerosis,* causes your arteries to thicken and impedes the flow of blood. This state of affairs also raises your blood pressure, forcing your heart to pump harder.

A chunk of plaque can break off and clog an artery, causing a heart attack or stroke. A stroke can also occur if blood clots form unexpectedly when you have greater-than-necessary amounts of clotting chemicals in your blood. These clots can get stuck in a blood vessel that feeds your brain (stroke), in a deep vessel running from your limbs to your heart (deep-vein thrombosis), in your lungs (pulmonary embolism), or in your heart (heart attack). All in all, your blood, blood vessels, and heart make up your *cardiovascular system,* and a problem in one area usually leads to trouble in another.

To avoid blood problems, doctors aim to keep your total cholesterol, LDL ('bad' cholesterol), and triglyceride levels low and keep your HDL ('good' cholesterol) levels high. This advice is important for anyone who's concerned about staying heart-healthy. But, when the topic at hand is predicting cardio-vascular risks for women, forget what you've heard about total cholesterol as the main event. The focus is on your triglycerides – keep them low – and your HDL levels – keep them high (refer to Chapter 5 for more on triglycerides and HDL levels.) Here's what the medical community knows about the effects of hormone replacement therapy on your blood.

Unopposed oestrogen

A variety of studies indicate that oestrogen (used as a pill or patch) without progesterone can provide a variety of benefits. Oestrogen:

> ✔ **Decreases LDL levels:** Oestrogen helps to get rid of some of the 'bad' cholesterol that furs your arteries. It increases the amount of LDL your liver breaks down, so more LDL is purged from your circulation. Oestrogen pills are more effective than patches at this job, but both work over time.

✔ **Increases HDL levels:** HDL cholesterol carries excess fat out of your bloodstream and back to your liver for reprocessing.

✔ **Improves the metabolism of carbohydrates:** Your body gets help digesting sugars, which helps to lower your risk of diabetes.

✔ **Helps maintain healthy blood clotting:** Like Goldilocks, you want it just right. Blood clots protect you from bleeding, but if you clot too easily you can have a stroke or develop artery-clogging deposits.

By helping to maintain healthy triglyceride and cholesterol levels in your blood, oestrogen lowers your risk of developing atherosclerosis, which is a major cause of angina, stroke, heart attacks, and other problems.

You can only use unopposed oestrogen if you no longer have your uterus.

Oestrogen plus progestogen

Do you see all the wonderful benefits oestrogen can bring? Well, add progestogen and the scenery changes. When added to oestrogen in hormone replacement therapy, progestogen tends to muffle the benefits of oestrogen. But hormone replacement therapy does slightly improve blood cholesterol, raising HDL levels slightly and lowering LDL levels slightly. Women using hormone replacement therapy generally have better blood cholesterol levels than women who don't use any hormone treatment at all.

Healthy blood helps to make a healthy you.

Keeping the Pipes Clean: HRT and Your Blood Vessels

Your heart stays alive and receives nourishment via your *coronary arteries,* blood vessels that deliver oxygen to your heart muscles. If your coronary arteries get messed up, trouble is in store.

Hormones play a major role in maintaining healthy blood vessels, including your coronary arteries. Your hormone levels must have the right balance to keep your blood vessels open and blood flowing smoothly through them. In the following sections we make the heart and hormone connection.

Avoiding clogs

When your blood contains more 'bad' fat (LDL cholesterol) than your HDLs can comfortably haul away, some of the fat is deposited inside your blood vessels. Trouble begins when your coronary arteries get clogged with fat and a gunk known as *fibrinogen* (a substance that helps blood to clot). After a while, the accumulation forms a crust called *plaque* (fat plus other substances form the foundation, with calcium on top of the pile). As plaque builds, it narrows your blood vessels and constricts the flow of blood to your heart – atherosclerosis is the diagnosis at this point.

In the following sections we look at what the studies have to say about the benefits and harms of hormone replacement therapy on atherosclerosis.

Unopposed oestrogen

Oestrogen not only helps your body maintain a healthy and balanced cholesterol profile (see 'Skimming the Fat: HRT and Your Blood' earlier in this chapter). Oestrogen also shines up your blood vessels:

- ✔ **Protecting your coronary arteries from plaque build-up:** Oestrogen prevents thickening of your artery walls and keeps plaque deposits from forming.

- ✔ **Keeping your vessels dilated:** Oestrogen relaxes the vessel walls to optimise blood flow throughout your circulation.

- ✔ **Decreasing plaque formation:** Oestrogen helps to prevent inflammatory cells sticking to blood vessel walls and triggering the development of plaque.

Oestrogen plus progestogen

The jury is still out on whether adding progestogen to the equation diminishes oestrogen's positive effects on blood vessels. None of the studies that look at this question is thorough.

The Nurses' Health Study indicates that progestogen didn't alter oestrogen's beneficial effects, but a study on monkeys showed that progestogen added to oestrogen blocked blood vessel dilation.

Controlling the pressure

Hypertension (the medical term for high blood pressure), usually produces no symptoms – that's why people call it the silent killer. As its nickname implies, hypertension is serious stuff. *Blood pressure* refers to the force created in your blood vessels as your heart pumps blood through your body. When your blood pressure rises, your heart has to pump harder to move blood through the tensed-up vessels, putting the vessels under even more pressure. The increased pressure damages the walls of your arteries and starts the process of *atherosclerosis* (fat and other gunk build up on the walls of your arteries). (For more information on high blood pressure, refer to Chapter 5.)

High blood pressure is a killer because it forces your heart to work harder, and worsens *coronary heart disease* in which your blood vessels become hard and scarred with plaque, losing their flexibility.

Unopposed oestrogen

The benefits outlined in this section are based on a number of studies using oestrogen therapy alone in women with no uterus. Oestrogen can positively impact your blood pressure and the health of your blood vessels as it:

- ✔ **Dilates arteries and other blood vessels in your body:** When arteries become wider, blood flows more efficiently.

- ✔ **Enhances the release of nitric oxide:** The release of nitric oxide relaxes your blood vessels so that blood flows more smoothly.

- ✔ **Improves blood flow in your coronary arteries:** This benefit is shown when taking oestrogen via a pill that dissolves under your tongue, but this is not yet available in the UK.

Oestrogen plus progestogen

The medical community doesn't have much research to turn to when looking for the effects that taking oestrogen and progestogen has on hypertension.

Keeping a clear head

Several different types of stroke occur, but the one related to menopause and hormone replacement therapy is ischaemic stroke. *Ischaemic stroke* occurs when an obstruction in an artery restricts the flow of blood – and the oxygen the blood carries – to your brain. The obstruction is often a piece of plaque that has broken off from the wall of an artery or a thickened artery wall damaged due to atherosclerosis.

A stroke suffocates the part of the brain whose nourishment comes from that clogged artery, impairing the functions that part of the brain directs. Deprived of oxygen, the brain section can die, which leads to some type of permanent debilitation. Strokes occur suddenly and, generally, without warning. The first indication is usually the loss of some movement or speech difficulties.

Oestrogen is thought to lower your risk of stroke because it provides so much protection to your blood and blood vessels. Keeping your pipes clean and flexible allows blood to flow without obstruction to your brain, which lowers your risk of ischaemic stroke. Here's what the latest research says about hormone replacement therapy and stroke.

The Women's Health Initiative study found that the use of conjugated oestrogen and MPA progestogen increases the risk of stroke for women. During the first year of using this particular blend of HRT, the risk of *deep-vein thrombosis* (DVT – blood clots in veins that empty into the heart) and *pulmonary embolism* (blood clots in the lungs) triples in comparison with women who aren't using any form of HRT.

Although at first glance this statistic seems frighteningly high, you need to bear in mind that, under normal circumstances, deep-vein thrombosis affects only 4 out of 10,000 women. Tripling the figure means that 12 women out of 10,000 using this blend of HRT develop DVT. It sounds small and is all a matter of perspective – unless, of course, it happens to you. The increased risk of these dangerous blood clots is probably why the risk of stroke goes up with use of this type of HRT.

Unopposed oestrogen

Oestrogen is thought to lower your risk of stroke because of its protective effects on your blood vessels and your blood's ability to clot properly. Check out the 'Controlling the pressure' and 'Skimming the Fat: HRT and Your Blood' sections earlier in this chapter for the positive effects of HRT on your blood vessels and your blood's ability to clot. But studies are mixed in their findings, and some results show an increased risk of DVT and stroke even among women who use only oestrogen.

Oestrogen plus progestogen

Another large study, the Nurses' Health Study, also shows that hormone replacement therapy (oestrogen plus a progestogen) slightly increases the risk of stroke in the first two years of use. After two years, the risk seems to drop back down to a similar level to that of women not using HRT.

Oiling the Pump: HRT and Your Heart

The changes that menopause brings have a large impact on your heart, so it makes sense that hormone replacement therapy has a large effect, too. But even if you take HRT, it is important to follow a healthy diet and to exercise regularly as these factors are also important in maintaining a healthy heart and circulation.

Slowing the pace

A fluttering heart doesn't always signal new love. Many women experience heart *palpitations* (a pounding, racing heart) for the first time during the change.

Palpitations can indicate a variety of cardiovascular problems. Doctors always take palpitations seriously. If you have palpitations, check your symptoms with your general practitioner.

When your oestrogen levels drop, as they do during the change, your brain triggers an increased output of adrenaline in an attempt to spur on oestrogen production. Your heart's response to this adrenaline surge is to beat more rapidly.

The effects of HRT on heart palpitations aren't really on the radar screen of scientists investigating the benefits and harms of hormone replacement therapy. We do know that HRT reduces perimenopausal symptoms, and heart palpitations are considered symptoms (as long as they're not indicative of more serious cardiovascular problems).

Keeping away angina

Angina can feel like you have a weight on your chest. We know: You're already carrying the weight of the world on your shoulders, so is it any wonder that it slips to your chest during menopause? Everything else seems to droop, after all! Although some women feel angina even when they are at rest, most women feel the pressure only when they exercise.

You feel the pressure of angina because your heart isn't getting enough blood. When you exercise, spasms cause your coronary arteries to tighten, which restricts the flow of blood to your heart. In response, your heart screams to get your attention, and you feel chest pain or tight discomfort.

Oestrogen has a soothing effect on blood vessels and reduces spasms. However, doctors are advised not to prescribe HRT just to treat angina or to prevent coronary heart disease. In fact, HRT possibly increases the risk of coronary heart disease – including angina – during the first year of use.

An exception is in the treatment of a relatively rare condition known as *cardiac syndrome X*, which, like its name, is a bit of a mystery. The condition is diagnosed when you experience typical tight angina heart pain during exercise but have sparklingly clear coronary arteries with no narrowing or blockages. Most people with cardiac syndrome X are menopausal women with symptoms of oestrogen withdrawal such as hot flushes and night sweats. Researchers believe that cardiac syndrome X occurs when lack of oestrogen stops small blood vessels (capillaries) in the heart muscle from dilating during exercise, so that the normal rush of blood and oxygen supplies into the area does not occur. Oestrogen replacement therapy can reduce both menopausal symptoms and the number of angina attacks experienced.

Avoiding the big one

The medical name for a heart attack is *myocardial infarction* (sometimes abbreviated to MI). A heart attack occurs when a blockage forms in one or more of your coronary arteries. This blockage is usually a blood clot or a plaque deposit that breaks from a blood vessel, flows through the bloodstream, and ends up clogging an artery. Blockages can restrict blood flow to your heart and cause the death of heart tissue – in other words, a heart attack.

Unopposed oestrogen

Oestrogen improves blood flow in your coronary arteries as it dilates blood vessels, helping your body to continue to eliminate plaque inside your vessels, and maintaining healthy clotting.

Oestrogen plus progestogen

The WHI study shows that women using conjugated oestrogen plus MPA progestogen have a 29 per cent higher risk of a heart attack than those not using HRT. But, although the risk of having a heart attack increases, the incidence of dying from one doesn't. Based on this information, some doctors are removing patients from hormone replacement therapy. Other doctors are taking more of a wait-and-see attitude, especially given that these results are out of whack with a number of other studies.

If you pull together information from all the other scientific studies (excluding the WHI) that look at coronary heart disease, heart attack, and hormone replacement therapy, results show that coronary heart disease is lower among women using hormone replacement therapy. However, when researchers look deeper into the situation, they find that exercise and alcohol use are the real factors making the difference, not the hormone replacement therapy, so the results are far from definitive. Until more research into the effects of hormone replacement therapy and heart health is available, take your doctor's advice on whether or not HRT is likely to suit you.

Chapter 12

Balancing HRT and Breast Cancer

. . . .

In This Chapter

▶ Recognising your risks of breast cancer

▶ Debating the benefits of HRT and the risk of breast cancer

▶ Choosing an HRT regimen with breast cancer in mind

. . . .

*I*s hormone replacement therapy (HRT) a risky business in terms of breast cancer? Medical experts suspecting a link between oestrogen and breast cancer can draw on over 60 years worth of research into this topic. Reports place oestrogen at the scene of the crime time and again, but no conclusive evidence demonstrates absolutely that oestrogen is the guilty party. And, if oestrogen is one of the perpetrators, some researchers claim that it may not act alone. This chapter shows you what researchers know for sure and what they're pretty sure they don't know about HRT and the risk of breast cancer.

Beginning with Breast Basics

Breast tissue and fat are the two main components of your breast. You probably already know about the fat – a subject that needs no further explanation. But the breast tissue is a relative stranger that needs an introduction.

Breast tissue comes in neat little sections called *lobes*. Lobes are made up of smaller *lobules,* which act as the milk factories when you breastfeed. *Ducts* carry milk from the lobules to the nipple. Breast cancers tend to form in the lobules or in the ducts. Figure 12-1 illustrates the important parts of your breasts.

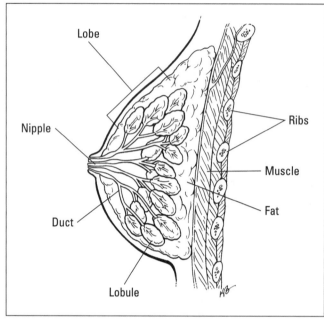

Figure 12-1:
The breast
and its com-
ponents.

Defining Breast Cancer

Whether breast cancer forms in the lobules or in the ducts, it begins when cells divide and grow at an abnormally fast rate. The cells morph into odd shapes and start clumping together to form cancerous (*malignant*) tumours.

What triggers this process? Researchers know that a *mutation* (a freak act of nature that affects the basic building blocks of cells) gets things going, but no one knows what makes the initial cells mutate. Most researchers believe that a *carcinogen* (a cancer-causing agent) in the environment serves as the trigger.

There are two main types of breast cancer and one condition that can lead to cancer:

✔ **Carcinoma *in situ*:** Technically, this is pre-cancer. *In situ* (which means *in place*) refers to the fact that the abnormal cells are still in their usual places and haven't spread beyond the lobule or duct in which they are found. Carcinoma *in situ* is like a breast cancer early-warning sign.

✔ **Invasive ductile cancer:** This type of cancer starts in the ducts and spreads to surrounding tissues.

✔ **Invasive lobular cancer:** This type of cancer starts in the lobules and spreads to surrounding tissues.

Both invasive ductile and invasive lobular cancers can move through the breast tissue into your blood vessels, gaining access to your entire body. When this happens, the cancer is said to *metastasise,* or spread.

Treating cancer is much easier when the cancer is confined to your breast, which is why early detection is so critical.

Taking Care of Your Breasts

You probably already know the importance of performing a monthly breast self-examination and having regular mammograms. In the following sections we explain why these two simple tests are so vital to your breast health.

Examining your breasts each month

Most breast cancers are first detected after women report unusual changes to their doctor. In the UK, breast cancer charities recommend that you remain breast aware, so that you get to know your own breasts and become familiar with how they look and feel. Report to your doctor without delay if you experience any of the following:

- ✔ Any change in the outline or shape of your breasts

- ✔ Any skin changes such as puckering or dimpling over a breast

- ✔ Any unusual discomfort or pain – especially if it keeps recurring

- ✔ Any lumps, thickening or bumpiness in one breast or armpit – especially if these are new or different from the other side

- ✔ Any change in a nipple, including change in position, turning inwards, unusual discharge, bleeding or rash that doesn't heal easily

The most common symptom of breast cancer during a self-examination is a hard, immovable lump in your breast, which may or may not feel tender. Sometimes the skin that stretches over the lump looks thick or indented; sometimes it looks dimpled like an orange peel. You may also notice that your nipple leaks a dark fluid or turns inward. If you notice any of these signs, contact your doctor straight away.

Try not to panic if you feel a lump. Nine out of ten breast lumps aren't cancerous but are fibrous nodules or fluid-filled cysts. Even though non-cancerous lumps are more common than cancerous lumps, all need urgent investigation as even doctors find it difficult to tell harmless lumps from cancerous lumps just using feel alone. For more information on breast conditions, take a look at *Women's Health For Dummies,* by Pamela Maraldo and the People's Medical Society (Wiley).

Making time for mammograms

Although you may see articles every year or so questioning the necessity of mammograms, most doctors say 'Just do it!' Mammograms are relatively painless, cost-effective, and fast.

Breast cancer is more common in older women, and regular breast screening of women over the age of 50 years reduces deaths from the disease. In the UK, women aged between 50 and 70 are invited to have a free National Health Service (NHS) mammogram every three years. You should accept this invitation and return for follow-ups if you are asked. The mammogram is as important a way of caring for your breasts as breast awareness, as it helps to detect unusual changes before you are aware of them yourself. The best chance of surviving breast cancer comes from early detection.

Some private health insurance companies offer mammography to women from the age of 40 years as part of their annual screen. Women under the age of 50 and who are at high risk of developing breast cancer are offered NHS mammography in certain areas of the UK but not others. The NHS has no national policy for this screening, as yet, as the evidence to show whether or not annual breast screening improves the successful treatment of high-risk women under the age of 50 is still under assessment.

Whether or not annual mammograms are ever offered on the NHS is a political question due to the cost of screening. Individuals who downplay the importance of annual screenings question whether mammography actually decreases the *death rate.* The more useful measure of the effectiveness of mammograms is whether regular mammograms increase the *detection rate* of new breast cancers – and they do! If you're a woman in your forties, having mammograms on a regular basis can reduce your chance of dying from breast cancer by as much as 17 per cent. For women between the ages of 50 and 69, regular mammograms can reduce deaths as much as 30 per cent.

Given a choice, most women would like to prevent long and arduous cancer treatments, which is the other important goal here. Early detection reduces the numbers of women who undergo drawn-out treatments for breast cancer. Mammograms detect cancers before they reach the size of a lump that you can feel. So, with today's mammogram technology, healthcare providers can identify cancer at an early stage, catching the cancer before it invades the bloodstream and gains access to other parts of your body. Early detection allows doctors to treat breast cancer with a relatively non-invasive and short course of treatment.

Establishing Oestrogen's Role

Although a great deal of controversy surrounds the 'whys' and 'hows', nearly everyone agrees that oestrogen plays a role in the development of breast cancer. Even the natural oestrogen in your body during your reproductive years increases your risk of breast cancer because it stimulates cell division in your breasts. Here are the things about oestrogen and menopause on which most experts agree:

✔ Oestrogen is a key promoter of breast cancer development. So controlling the oestrogen levels in your breast tissue may well lower your risk of breast cancer.

✔ The earlier you begin perimenopause and the shorter your reproductive cycle, the lower your risk of breast cancer because these factors decrease you total lifetime exposure to high levels of oestrogen.

✔ If you are overweight after menopause (gaining 20.4 kilograms (3 stone 3 pounds) or more since your 18th birthday or reaching 20 per cent over your target weight), this extra weight increases oestrogen levels in your body and can increase your risk of breast cancer. (In Chapter 18 we help you determine your ideal weight.)

Although being overweight does not increase the risk of breast cancer in pre-menopausal women, extra weight does put you at risk of other health problems. Try to lose as much excess fat as possible – whatever your age.

Assessing Your Risk of Breast Cancer

A woman over the age of 40 already has two of the biggest risk factors for breast cancer: Female gender and increasing age. Unless you discover the Fountain of Youth, both risks are realistically unavoidable.

Breast-cancer risk continues to rise after menopause, regardless of whether you take hormones. But a number of other factors can also increase your risk of breast cancer. Some are controllable; and some aren't.

Recognising risks you can't control

Frustratingly, some breast-cancer risk factors are out of your control. Even your own oestrogen appears to heighten your breast-cancer risks (see the 'Establishing Oestrogen's Role' section earlier in this chapter). This section lists the other risks that you can't do anything about.

> ✔ **Age:** The older you get, the greater your risk of breast cancer. When you're younger than 40, your risk of breast cancer is quite low. But, after 40, your breast-cancer risk increases until the age of 80. After that, we have good news – when you hit 80, your risk of breast cancer actually decreases a bit, as we show in Figure 12-2.

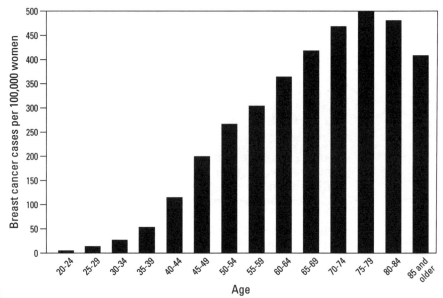

Figure 12-2: Age as a risk factor for breast cancer.

> ✔ **Breast density:** Breasts with more breast tissue than fat tissue are comparatively more dense when viewed on a mammogram. At least one major health study shows that the denser your breast tissue, the greater your risk of cancer, but unfortunately, detecting small tumours in dense breast tissue is less easy than detecting them in fatty tissue.

> ✔ **Ethnicity:** White women tend to have a higher risk of breast cancer than black women, probably due to different cultures and lifestyles, such as the number of children you have and at what age. Ashkenazi Jews and Icelandic women are at greater risk of breast cancer than women from

some other cultures. No one knows exactly why these women are at higher risk, but some evidence shows that they are more likely to inherit genes associated with a higher risk of breast cancer, such as *BRCA1* and *BRCA2* (which we discuss next).

✔ **Genetics:** If someone in your immediate family – mother or sister – has breast cancer, your risk of breast cancer almost doubles. If both your mum and a sister have breast cancer, your risk is about two and a half times greater than the risk of a woman without breast cancer in her family.

If you're worried about your family history of breast cancer, you may want to take genetic tests that look for two genetic mutations – *BRCA1* and *BRCA2* – that leave you more susceptible to breast cancer. However, only about 5–10 per cent of breast cancers come from inherited genetic mutations.

The letters BRCA stand for *breast cancer*. *BRCA1* is a genetic mutation found in people with a family history of ovarian and breast cancer. *BRCA2* is a genetic mutation found in people with a family history of male and female breast cancer. Only about 50–60 per cent of women with these genes actually get breast cancer, and remember that these genes only account for 5–10 per cent of all breast cancer cases.

The genetic tests are easy, but dealing with the results is more complicated. Before having the test, consider what you want to do with the results. Will it simply cause you greater anxiety? Also, find out what measures are in place to guarantee confidentiality so that the results are available to you alone and not to insurance companies or other parties.

✔ **Location of fat in your body:** This may sound strange, and you can't really do anything about it, but studies show that if you wear your fat around your waist (apple-shape), your risk of breast cancer is about six times higher than for a woman who wears her fat around her hips, thighs, and buttocks (pear-shape).

✔ **Menstrual history:** The later you begin your menstrual cycle and the earlier you reach the menopause, the lower your risk of breast cancer. Presumably, your risk of breast cancer is tied to the amount of oestrogen you generate during your lifetime.

✔ **'Precancerous' breast tumours:** Receiving a diagnosis of abnormal cell growth, carcinoma *in situ,* for example, increases your risk of breast cancer. (Check out the 'Defining Breast Cancer' section earlier in this chapter for more on carcinoma *in situ.*)

What if you've already had breast cancer?

If you've had breast cancer in one breast, you're at greater risk of developing cancer in the other breast. Women with a history of ovarian or uterine cancer are also at slightly greater risk of breast cancer.

If you have experience of breast cancer, you and your doctor are likely to decide that HRT is out of the question for you. In fact, the literature that comes with oestrogen medications tells doctors not to use them to treat women with previous or existing breast cancers. Although HRT is not right for you, medications such as SERMs are available to prevent postmenopausal osteoporosis (although they do not reduce menopausal hot flushes). (For more information on SERMs, see Chapter 10. For more information on reducing menopausal symptoms without HRT, see Chapters 16 to 19).

Fibrocystic breast disease, a condition in which you develop little lumps in your breast tissue (usually seven to ten days before your period), does *not* increase your risk of breast cancer. (For more information on fibrocystic condition of the breast, read *Women's Health For Dummies,* by Pamela Maraldo and the People's Medical Society (Wiley).)

Realising the risks you can control

Don't feel forlorn – you can control a lot of the risks associated with breast cancer. To improve your odds and take control of these factors, try evaluating your current lifestyle for behaviours that carry high breast-cancer risks. Check out the following list – if you're already living a 'breast-healthy' lifestyle, well done. Give yourself a pat on the back!

- ✔ **Alcohol consumption:** Having more than three units of alcohol a week raises your risk of breast cancer. This fact holds true whether you're taking hormone replacement therapy (HRT) or not, but is especially true if you take the conjugated equine form of oestrogen. Alcohol raises the level of the oestrone type of oestrogen in your body.

 (For more info about conjugated equine oestrogen, check out the 'Choosing your HRT regimen with breast cancer in mind' section later in this chapter. And for more on all forms of oestrogens used in HRT, take a look at Chapter 10.)

- ✔ **Antioxidants:** Vitamins A, C, E, carotenoids, selenium, and glutathione are antioxidants that protect your body from premature ageing and cancer (see Chapter 18 for more on antioxidants). When taken during menopause, these antioxidants help to lower the risk of breast cancer.

✔ **Dietary fat:** This is a bit controversial as some studies indicate that high-fat diets increase your risk, while other studies are inconclusive, and yet others show that fat has no bearing on the risk of breast cancer. The studies that show a high-fat diet increases your risk suggest that fat shouldn't make up more than 20 per cent of your daily calories (so if, for example, you eat 2,000 calories a day, only 400 calories are fat) – and that's pretty unpalatable.

The type of fat you eat also affects your risk. *Saturated fats* (the types of fat that you find in animal products such as red meat and cheese) raise your risk of breast cancer. Animal fats also introduce a number of by-products into your diet that come from the animals' environment, such as pesticides and antibiotics, which are concentrated in the animal fat. This is less of a problem if you only eat organic meat.

✔ **Exercise:** Studies that tracked patients for more than ten years show that cancer deaths decrease as women raise their activity levels.

✔ **Pregnancy:** Women who experience at least one pregnancy have a lower risk of breast cancer during their *lifetime* than women who never get pregnant. But you have to read the fine print that accompanies this risk factor because you actually have a slightly higher risk of breast cancer during the ten years immediately following the birth. After ten years or so, your risk of breast cancer drops so that women with one child have a lower risk of breast cancer than women who never bear a child. In general, the more babies you have, the lower your lifetime risk of breast cancer. Breastfeeding for a total of at least one year (spread over all your babies) appears to protect against breast cancer, too.

✔ **Weight gain/obesity:** Gaining more than 20.4 kilograms (3 stone 3 pounds) during your adult life increases your risk of breast cancer after the menopause. Breast cancer is linked to higher levels of oestrogen (especially the *oestrone* oestrogen found in fat). Obese women (who weigh 20 per cent more than their target weight) are also at greater risk because they have about 40 per cent more oestrogen on board than non-obese women. (Check out Chapter 18 for additional information on weight-related issues.)

Evaluating the Facts about HRT Risks

Everywhere you turn, there are conflicting stories about the risks of breast cancer as a result of taking hormone replacement therapy (HRT). Individuals and groups within the medical community provide different opinions depending on whom you talk to. The source of conflict among experts essentially comes down to the reliability of results from studies testing the breast-cancer/HRT connection. Some studies use small groups when large groups are more reliable, while those based on large numbers of women rely on observations or participant's memories instead of objective tests. And the type of HRT tested also varies from study to study. So, unravelling the connections is often difficult and fraught with disagreement.

If, as Paul Simon sings, there are 50 ways to leave a lover, there are thousands of ways to disagree with research results. In the following sections, we attempt to present both sides of the debate concerning hormone replacement therapy and breast-cancer risk.

Argument: Avoid hormone replacement therapy to avoid breast cancer

The research results that experts rely on to warn of the dangers associated with oestrogen and breast cancer include:

- ✔ Women whose uterus and ovaries have been surgically removed before age 40 (and, therefore, stop producing oestrogen before 40 years of age) have a lower incidence of breast cancer. Because your body's own oestrogen contributes to the risk of breast cancer, hormone replacement therapy will too.

Knowing for sure: Tests for breast cancer

If you find a lump in your breast, your doctor refers you to a specialist breast clinic where you see a specialist as soon as possible – ideally within two weeks. The specialist uses several ways to see whether a lump contains cancer cells. The type of test your doctor uses depends on the size of the lump and its location.

- ✔ **Fine-needle aspiration:** This procedure involves sticking a tiny needle into your lump, sucking out a few cells and/or fluid for examination.

- ✔ **Needle core biopsy:** Because the doctor uses a bigger needle for this test, he or she also uses a local anaesthetic to numb the area. The doctor sticks the needle into the suspected problem area, to remove a sample of breast tissue.

- ✔ **Open biopsy:** This surgical procedure is performed under a general anaesthetic. The doctor makes a small incision and removes part of the lump or the entire lump.

Biopsy specimens removed during these procedures are sent straight off to a laboratory, where scientists mount the specimens on glass slides, stain the specimens, and examine them under a microscope to see whether they contain cancer cells.

✔ The biggest and best randomised, controlled study to date, is the Women's Health Initiative (WHI) study, which clearly shows that women taking conjugated oestrogen with MPA progestogen are at increased risk of breast cancer after using it for over five years. Also, it seems that the longer you take HRT, the greater your risk. (For more information on different types of oestrogen and progestogen used in HRT, check out Chapter 10.)

✔ The Million Women Study is an observational study of a million women, which shows that women taking conjugated equine oestrogens, or oestradiol, or oestrogen-progestogen combinations (sequential and continuous), or tibolone (a synthetic hormone with both oestrogen and progestogen actions) for several years have an increased risk of breast cancer, with no difference in risk between the different routes of administration.

The doctors occupying this camp also argue that using less risky, non-HRT drugs are available to treat most of the conditions that HRT regimens help (check out Chapter 17 for more on these medications).

Argument: The benefits of HRT outweigh the risks

Experts who believe that HRT benefits outweigh the risks of breast cancer have this to say:

✔ Several studies report no increase in the risk of breast cancer in women who use oestrogen at one time or another.

✔ Among women who do not use HRT, the risk of breast cancer is highest in the post-menopausal years. This shows that the incidence of breast cancer rises as you get older, even if you don't use HRT.

✔ Some studies suggest that higher rates of breast cancer occur only in women who both take oestrogen and also drink alcohol.

✔ If you compare women on HRT with those not on HRT, the death rates from breast cancer are similar. One may expect a higher death rate in women who use HRT if it causes breast cancer.

✔ A higher percentage of low-grade, less aggressive breast cancers exists among women who take HRT versus those who don't. If HRT promotes breast cancer, it promotes a less aggressive form.

Interpreting the evidence

The previous sections tell the story of HRT and the risk of breast cancer as the medical establishment understands it today. Research continues, and a less confusing conclusion may prevail in years to come.

At the moment, the UK's Committee on Safety of Medicines (CSM) estimates that using *all* types of HRT, including tibolone, increases the risk of breast cancer within one to two years of starting treatment. The increased risk relates to the length of HRT use, but not the age at which you start it, and this excess risk disappears within about five years of stopping treatment.

For women aged 50–64 years and not using HRT, around 14 out of 1,000 develop breast cancer every five years. In those taking *oestrogen-only* HRT for five years, an extra 1.5 cases of breast cancer is diagnosed per 1,000 women. In those using *combined* HRT for 5 years, an extra 6 cases of breast cancer is diagnosed per 1,000 women.

If we include older women, who have a higher risk of breast cancer, and widen the age range to 50–79 years, then around 31 out of every 1,000 women not using HRT is diagnosed with breast cancer every five years. In those using *oestrogen-only* HRT for 5 years, no extra cases are diagnosed, but in those using *combined* HRT for 5 years, an extra 4 cases of breast cancer develops per 1,000 women.

Tibolone increases the risk of breast cancer but to a lesser extent than *combined* HRT.

Of course, the HRT choice is yours. But here are a few things to think about when reviewing all the evidence:

- ✔ **What are your individual health risks?** If you or any of your family members have osteoporosis or dementia, you may want to think seriously about taking HRT. If you have a family history of breast cancer, then caution is wise. Breast cancer is a terrible disease, but sometimes, people underestimate the consequences of osteoporosis, which HRT can lessen, and dementia, which HRT may impede, although HRT is not indicated first-line for these uses.

- ✔ **What can you live with?** What concessions are you willing to make? Combating osteoporosis requires a healthy diet and a regular exercise programme, often in combination with medication. Are you able to stay on track if you have to take medication and increase your exercise to fight osteoporosis? Everyone agrees that oestrogen relieves perimenopausal symptoms such as hot flushes and other symptoms that we discuss in Chapter 3. Can you live with these symptoms? Cancer scares all of us, no matter how small the risk. Considering the evidence about the links between HRT and the risk of breast cancer, how do you evaluate your risk?

✔ **What do you fear most?** Some people dread getting Alzheimer's disease; some fear having a heart attack; and others worry about cancer. Use these opinions when considering your alternatives.

As research results don't provide an obvious choice concerning HRT, you need to rely on your own health goals and interpretation of the research results.

Finding the Right HRT Programme for You

Over the years, the medical establishment has reached a consensus on the need for different hormone replacement therapy (HRT) regimens because women have different hormone profiles, menopausal symptoms, and medical conditions. And certain types of oestrogen result in a higher risk of breast cancer than others. In the case of HRT, one size will not fit all.

Reading your alphabet soup: Results from the WHI and MAWS on HRT and BC

The Women's Health Initiative (WHI) trial from 2002, is one of the new and improved randomised, controlled studies that includes tens of thousands of women (a huge study by anyone's standards). The WHI researchers also use highly sophisticated techniques to make sure that the study results aren't biased in terms of the type of women chosen to participate. Women of all ages, ethnicities, medical histories, and so forth took part. The results provide loads of hard facts about the use of the most commonly prescribed HRT regimen in the US (although this regimen is less common in the UK).

And here's the problem: You can't necessarily generalise and say that these results are the hard and fast facts about *all the different HRT products* currently prescribed in the UK. We know that different types of oestrogen and progesterone produce different effects. Conjugated oestrogens have different effects than oestradiol oestrogen, and pills work differently than patches (for the details on the differences, turn to Chapter 10).

The Million Women Study (MAWS) from 2003 involves over a million women, all from the UK, but is not a randomised, controlled trial – it's a multi-centre population study in which women attending for breast screening answer questions about their health and use of HRT and are then followed up to see if they develop breast cancer. Even so, it suggests that current use of HRT is associated with an increased risk of breast cancer, and the effect is substantially greater for oestrogen-progestogen combinations than other types of HRT.

Discussing HRT and breast cancer with your doctor

Because no clear-cut answers exist about whether HRT raises your risk of breast cancer, most doctors try to advise you about the benefits and potential risks concerning HRT instead of simply writing a prescription and sending you on your way. If your doctor doesn't present you with a balanced comparison of the benefits and risks associated with HRT, ask him or her to discuss these with you. The HRT decision isn't one to take lightly, and your doctor's role is to spend time making you feel comfortable about your choices.

Choosing your HRT regimen with breast cancer in mind

The Women's Health Initiative (WHI) study suggests that *conjugated equine oestrogen,* which is made from the urine of pregnant horses, is the type of oestrogen most likely to increase the risk of breast cancer. (For more information on the different forms of oestrogen used in HRT, refer to Chapter 10.) This type of oestrogen gives you much higher levels of *oestrone* (the inactive form of oestrogen) and long-lasting oestrogens that seem to bond stronger and longer to the oestrogen receptors in the breast.

But to be fair, conjugated equine oestrogen is the most widely used in the US, and is therefore the most widely studied form of oestrogen, which may explain why this type of oestrogen is more closely related to breast cancer than other forms.

Evidence from the UK Million Women Study suggests that all types of HRT increase the risk of breast cancer within 1–2 years of starting treatment, and that the effect is substantially greater for oestrogen-progestogen combinations than for other types of HRT.

Take a close look at yourself when you answer the question 'Is HRT right for me?' The role of HRT in breast cancer is still not answered fully. You need to review all the available information on breast cancer and HRT with your doctor, and then consider your own medical issues and family history.

Considering the alternatives

If you smoke or use alcohol daily, if you're obese, or if you have breast cancer in your immediate family, you definitely need to discuss HRT with your doctor and discuss all the possible alternatives to hormone replacement therapy. Think about your medical risks, your values, and your preferences in making your decision.

Chapter 13

Talking About HRT and Other Cancer Risks

. . . .

In This Chapter

▶ Recognising how hormone therapy affects cancers of your reproductive and digestive tract

▶ Examining screening procedures and tests

▶ Considering the cancer-related benefits and risks of HRT

. . . .

*H*ormone replacement therapy (HRT) has links with all kinds of non-breast cancers including urinary, digestive, and reproductive organs – and not all links are bad. In some cases, HRT actually seems to lower the risk of cancer. In other cases, HRT may increase the risk of some cancers. In yet other cases, HRT is thought to have absolutely no effect.

In this chapter we look at cervical, colon (or more accurately colorectal), endometrial (uterine), and ovarian cancers. We introduce the symptoms of each of these cancers, review the screening procedures and tests used to diagnose them, and discuss the role (or lack thereof) that HRT plays in connection with each cancer.

What about breast cancer? Well, because of all the issues that surround this topic, it gets an entire chapter of its own – refer to Chapter 12 for more information.

Colorectal Cancer

The colon and rectum are the last stops on your digestive tract before waste moves out of your body. The first six feet or so of your large intestine is called the *colon;* the last six inches is called the *rectum.* If you're wondering how your body holds six feet of tubing (not to mention the 10 or 11 feet of small intestines that come before it), take a look at Figure 13-1, which shows the location of the colon and rectum.

Although commonly known as colon cancer, the proper name for this type of cancer is *colorectal cancer* as it can occur in the colon or the rectum. Some people refer to it as bowel cancer.

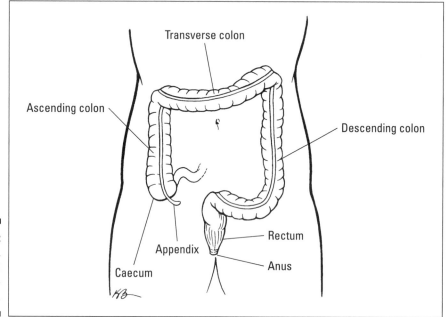

Figure 13-1:
The colon, rectum, and other connections.

Colorectal cancer is a slow-growing cancer that begins as a *polyp* (a small growth) on the mucous lining (*mucosa*) of the colon, as shown in Figure 13-2. Polyps can show up in the colon and remain perfectly harmless (asking why is like asking cats why they pounce; they just do). But some polyps have the potential to turn cancerous.

Colorectal cancer is one of the most common cancers and is the third leading cause of cancer death (after lung and breast cancer) of women in the UK. Over 90 per cent of cases of colorectal cancer are found in people over 50 years of age. Colorectal cancer is easily detectable, and you can easily prevent it through healthy lifestyle choices and having regular check-ups.

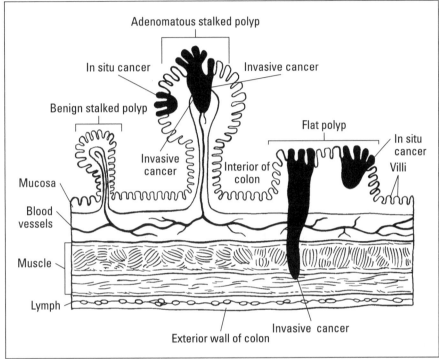

Figure 13-2: Polyps in the colon may become cancerous.

Recognising the signs

Rectal bleeding and bloody stools are the most common symptoms of colorectal cancer. Additional symptoms include a change in bowel habit, (diarrhoea, constipation, skinny stools) frequent gas pains, and feeling like you can't completely pass a stool. Some people with this disease lose weight, feel fatigued, or develop *anaemia* (a condition in which you don't have enough red blood cells to carry oxygen around your body).

Finding out for sure: Screenings and tests

When your doctor checks you out for colorectal cancer, he or she looks for cancer *and* polyps on the lining of your colon. Removing any polyps removes some of your future cancer risk.

A number of screening procedures reduce your risk of colon cancer. Having regular screening is the number-one way to reduce your risk of colorectal cancer.

Here's why catching polyps early is so important: When colorectal cancer is found before it spreads to other areas of the body, the survival rate is 90 per cent. When colorectal cancer spreads, long-term survival rates drop to 9 per cent. So getting regular screenings after you turn 50 is well worth the effort.

Generally doctors start out with minimally invasive screening procedures, such as a digital examination and faecal occult blood test, (which we explain next), and then move on to more invasive procedures only when initial results warrant additional tests. The following tests are generally your first line of defence:

- ✔ **Digital rectal examination:** This test is probably the part of your medical check-up that you look forward to the least. Your doctor inserts a gloved finger into your rectum to check for lumps, bumps, and other changes in the rectum.

- ✔ **Faecal occult blood (FOB) test:** This test is a bit messy, but it is really essential. Some of the newer tests look like a home pregnancy kit – a piece of paper turns a different colour if your sample has blood in it. During your examination, your doctor takes a sample and places it on a test card. You and your doctor can see the results of this test immediately. People who have two-yearly FOB screening are 15 per cent less likely to die from colorectal cancer than those not screened. A bowel cancer screening programme is now phasing in throughout England and Scotland, and will be extended to Wales and Northern Ireland in 2009. If you are 60 years or over, this screening programme offers to send FOB test kits to your own home every two years. You send them back to a laboratory for analysis.

If blood is in your stool or your doctor feels something suspicious during the digital exam, he or she may perform one of the following procedures to check things out further:

- ✔ **Colonoscopy:** You normally have a mild sedative before this test. During the test, your doctor inserts a long, thin, flexible scope into your colon, which allows him or her to carefully examine the walls of your colon and rectum (yes, all six feet or so). Your doctor may even take pictures of your colon wall and any polyps. Usually your doctor then removes any polyps and sends them to a laboratory, where scientists test them for evidence of cancer.

- ✔ **Sigmoidoscopy:** You normally have a sedative before this test. Your doctor inserts a short, thin, flexible scope about 10 to 12 inches into your rectum, through which he or she can see any polyps or damaged areas in the last section of your colon and take a sample if necessary.

✔ **Barium enema:** This procedure involves flushing the bowel with a barium solution before taking a series of X-rays of your colon and rectum. The barium highlights your colon, particularly any polyps and growths. Barium enemas are rarely used now. Most doctors perform a colonoscopy or sigmoidoscopy instead to directly visualise the bowel walls and take any necessary biopsies.

Determining the role of HRT

For reasons unknown (although most researchers suspect that oestrogen plays the heroic role here), hormone replacement therapy (HRT) lowers your risk of colon cancer. In fact, you reduce your risk of colon cancer by more than one-third when you take HRT.

The risk reduction exists only when you are on HRT. The protection diminishes after you stop taking HRT.

Assessing your risks

Some of the factors that raise your risk of colorectal cancer are:

✔ **Age:** Over 90 per cent of people with colorectal cancer are over the age of 50. With each decade after 50, your risk doubles.

✔ **Diet:** Eating red meat or processed meat frequently (once a day) can double your risk of colon cancer. Animal fat is one culprit here, as toxins tend to gather in it. If the animal you're eating was exposed to pesticides or other toxins before it became dinner, you get those poisons when you eat it. The main risk is in cooking meat at high temperatures or for long durations, which produces cancer-causing chemicals known as heterocyclic amines.

✔ **Family history:** Genetics play a role in colorectal cancer (and many other cancers as well). If you have one or more family members with colon cancer, your risk doubles.

A couple of genetic syndromes bump up your chance for colorectal cancer, but they're quite rare. These syndromes include *familial adenomatous polyposis* and *hereditary nonpolyposis colorectal cancer*.

✔ **Lifestyle:** Is going from the couch to the freezer to grab a bowl of icecream your idea of a brisk walk? If so, listen carefully: You can cut your risk of colorectal cancer in half if you get out and exercise. Whether you cycle, jog, or simply walk (no, your couch-to-freezer regimen doesn't count), you lower your risk. Turn to Chapter 19 for more on exercising your way to better health.

Endometrial (Uterine) Cancer

Cancer of the uterus is usually called *endometrial cancer* as it usually starts in the *endometrium* – the lining of the uterus. Take a look at Figure 13-3 to see the uterus and related organs.

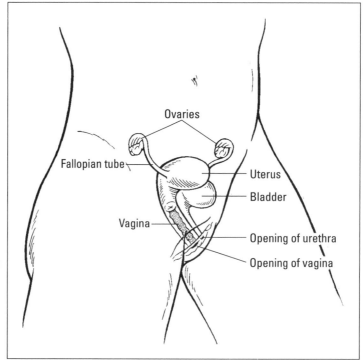

Figure 13-3: The female reproductive organs.

In the UK, endometrial cancer is the second most common cancer of the female genital tract (after cancer of the ovaries) and is the fifth most common female cancer overall. Endometrial cancer is readily detected – 75 per cent of cases are caught before the cancer moves beyond the uterus – and treatment is effective.

Your endometrium is responsive to changes in hormone levels. Like many cancers, endometrial cancer occurs when mutant cancer cells grow abnormally fast. Too high a level of oestrogen or continued high levels of oestrogen over a sustained period of time cause cells in the endometrium to continue to multiply. If mutant cancer cells are among those normal endometrial cells, the oestrogen stimulates cell growth and allows the cancer cells to multiply along with the normal cells. Developing the occasional cancer cell is usually not a problem because it gets flushed away during your period, so it doesn't have a chance to proliferate. But, with high levels of oestrogen (stimulating cell growth), these cancer cells can multiply more rapidly and take hold.

If you don't have a uterus because you've had a hysterectomy, you don't need to worry about endometrial cancer because you don't have any endometrial tissue.

Recognising the signs

Most cases of endometrial cancer are caught early enough to cure because the symptoms are so obvious. Any of the following symptoms are a signal to see your doctor:

- ✔ Bleeding after menopause
- ✔ Irregular vaginal bleeding
- ✔ Unusual spotting between periods

Pain and cramping are generally *not* an early symptom of this type of endometrial cancer. (But, after endometrial cancer develops, it can invade the blood vessels and spread to other organs causing this type of pain.) Some women experience no symptoms of endometrial cancer at all.

Finding out for sure: Tests

A number of tests can identify endometrial cancer:

- ✔ **Dilation and curettage:** Often referred to as a *D&C,* this test involves scraping tissue from the lining of the uterus for examination. Doctors usually perform the D&C procedure while you are under a general anaesthetic in an operating theatre.

- ✔ **Endometrial aspiration or biopsy:** With this test, your doctor removes a tissue sample from the lining of your uterus for examination. Endometrial aspirations are carried out in out-patient clinics. The procedure is a bit like having a smear test, and usually you do not need any painkilling medication beyond ibuprofen.

- ✔ **Hysteroscopy:** This test involves your doctor inserting a special microscope into your uterus to examine the lining – you are usually under anaesthesia in an operating theatre for this procedure.

Looking at the life of the endometrium

When you have your period, the surface of the *endometrium* (the lining of the uterus) sloughs off, leaving behind just a thin layer of endometrial cells. At the end of your period, your ovaries bump up the level of oestrogen production.

In response to this higher level of oestrogen, your endometrium thickens. You then ovulate, at which time your ovaries produce even higher levels of oestrogen along with progesterone.

The oestrogen continues to tell your endometrium to grow thicker, and the progesterone causes it to develop blood vessels and store nutrients for nurturing a fertilised egg.

If no fertilised egg arrives, the progesterone and oestrogen levels drop, your period begins, and you slough off much of the endometrium. If the egg is fertilised, you continue to produce high levels of progesterone.

✔ **Ultrasound:** Using sound waves, your doctor can create images of your uterus lining with this test. Ultrasounds are carried out in out-patient clinics and are relatively painless. An ultrasound wand is inserted into the vagina so that the technician can get a clear view of your uterus and its lining.

Determining the role of HRT

The higher the dose of oestrogen in your HRT and the longer the duration of your high oestrogen levels, the higher the risk of developing cancer in your uterus.

In the 1970s, after women had taken oestrogen replacement therapy without a *progestogen* (a synthetic form of progesterone) for years, medical experts noticed that the incidence of endometrial cancer was three to eight times higher among women taking oestrogen compared with women not taking it.

Doctors began to realise that, without a progestogen, the lining of the uterus continues to thicken unchecked. So now, hormone replacement therapy includes a progestogen to routinely flush the lining of the uterus through vaginal bleeding (cyclical hormone therapy) or to keep the lining from growing (continuous hormone therapy). Chapter 10 provides more information on the different types of hormone replacement therapy.

If you don't have a uterus because you've had a hysterectomy, you don't need a progestogen in your hormone therapy to balance the oestrogen to avoid endometrial cancer.

Assessing your risks

Because an imbalance in hormones (particularly oestrogen and progesterone) increases your risk of endometrial cancer, things that alter your hormone levels can raise your risk:

- **Age:** Over 95 per cent of women with endometrial cancer are over 40 years of age. The rate of endometrial cancer rises between the ages of 40 and 70, and then drops around age 80.

- **Obesity:** Fat tissue produces oestrogen. Women who are 20 per cent over their ideal weight walk around with persistently high levels of oestrogen because their body fat produces it. Fat is the primary producer of oestrogen in women after menopause. (For more on weight-related issues, see Chapters 18 and 19.)

  If you're obese, losing weight reduces your risk of endometrial cancer.

- **Oestrogen:** Taking oestrogen replacement therapy without a progestogen increases your risk of endometrial cancer. But at least one study shows that women who use a combination of oestrogen and progestogen have a lower risk of endometrial cancer than women who do not use HRT at all.

Women who have never had a pregnancy have not experienced long periods of high progesterone levels. So obese women with no prior pregnancies are at an even higher risk of endometrial cancer.

Birth-control pills *lower* your risk of endometrial cancer. Women who use the pill for more than two years halve their risk, while women who use the pill for more than five years have an 80 per cent lower risk compared with women not using the pill.

Cancers Unaffected by HRT

In this section we mention a few other cancers of the female persuasion. Hormone replacement therapy (HRT) has no known effects on your risk of developing these cancers or your ability to recover from them, but we think that a book that addresses health issues facing menopausal women is incomplete without at least discussing these cancers.

Cervical cancer

Cervical cancer is the same thing as cancer of the cervix. A *cervical smear* usually detects this form of cancer quite early. Certain types of genital wart virus (human papilloma viruses) are associated with cervical cancer, so practising safe sex can prevent it. The types of wart virus associated with cervical cancer do not cause visible genital warts, so don't panic if you need treatment for visible genital warts.

HRT is not known to have any impact on cervical cancer.

Ovarian cancer

The *ovaries* hold your *oocytes* (seeds that develop into eggs over the course of your reproductive years) and produce sex hormones throughout your life. Take a look at Figure 13-3 to locate the ovaries. Ovarian cancer originates from cells in the ovary – both the egg-making cells and the lining of the ovary.

Cancer of the ovaries (*ovarian cancer*) kills silently. Few tangible symptoms warn women of this disease until the tumour spreads beyond the ovary. Even in the later stages of the disease, the symptoms are pretty general – bloating, nausea, vomiting, constipation, and frequent urination. A lot of things can cause these problems – a bad piece of fish, too much wine, the flu, you name it. Ovarian cancer is deadly, and is the most common cancer of the female genital tract. Nearly 7,000 cases are diagnosed in the UK each year.

Some researchers suggest that ovarian cancer is related to frequency of ovulation during your lifetime. Every time you ovulate, you get a little tear in the ovary wall. The cells of your ovary divide rapidly to repair the tear and this monthly, rapid cell division is perhaps the source of ovarian cancer. Given this explanation, women who take birth-control pills (the old-time high-dose pills or newer low-dose pills) may actually have a lower risk of ovarian cancer because the pill suppresses ovulation.

If you've had no pregnancies, you may have a higher risk of ovarian cancer than women who have had babies, or pregnancies lasting beyond 24 weeks, simply because you don't experience prolonged periods of time during which you don't ovulate.

Recognising the signs

Most of the symptoms of ovarian cancer are quite generic – in other words, they apply to any number of conditions. Many women first notice bloating in their abdomen, which is easy to confuse with some of the symptoms of pre-menstrual syndrome. Other women experience nausea, vomiting, or gas that just won't go away despite changes in diet. Frequent urination and constipation are also possible symptoms as are abdominal or pelvic pain. The problem is that the symptoms usually aren't present until the disease enters an advanced stage.

Finding out for sure: Tests

If you experience any of the symptoms listed in the 'Recognising the signs' section, ask your doctor for a pelvic examination and a blood test that looks for the presence of CA125. *CA125* is an ovarian cancer *antigen*, meaning a substance that causes the body to fight ovarian cancer. If your CA125 levels are high, you may have ovarian cancer. Unfortunately determining the meaning of high CA125 levels is tricky. Sometimes high levels show up if you have endometriosis, ovarian cysts, or fibroids, or if you're pregnant. Because this test is not specifically helpful as a specific screening or diagnostic test for ovarian cancer, some doctors don't use it.

Just because your CA125 levels aren't elevated doesn't necessarily mean you definitely don't have ovarian cancer – 20–30 per cent of women with ovarian cancer don't have elevated CA125 levels. Likewise, having elevated CA125 levels doesn't mean that you absolutely do have ovarian cancer, but does provide a reason to further explore the cause of the results.

As the symptoms of ovarian cancer are so disarming and the disease is so deadly, CA125 provides doctors with one point of information in trying to diagnose this disease early. Plus, a CA125 test may identify more *benign* (not cancerous) medical conditions such as endometriosis and fibroids. All in all, if you're having symptoms, taking this test is a good idea. Medical types use a variety of other tests (in addition to a pelvic examination and CA125 test) in their attempts to detect ovarian cancer:

- ✔ **CAT scan:** The *CAT* here stands for *computerised axial tomography.* This procedure lets your doctor see a graphical image of your ovaries to check for tumours.

- ✔ **Laparoscopy:** This is a minor surgical procedure in which your doctor makes a tiny incision in your belly button and inserts a scope to get a better view of your ovaries. This examination is done under a general anaesthetic in an operating room on an out-patient basis.

- ✔ **Pelvic ultrasound:** With this exam, the doctor or technician inserts a sounding device into your vagina to produce an image (a *sonogram*) of your ovaries and identify tumours whether they are cystic (filled with fluid) or solid.

Determining the role of hormones

The UK Committee on Safety of Medicines estimates that 3 in every 1,000 women aged 50–69 years who are **not** using HRT develop ovarian cancer over five years, rising to 4 in every 1,000 women (one extra case) in those using oestrogen-only HRT. Recent research suggests that the risk of ovarian cancer is possibly even higher than this.

Birth-control pills may reduce your risks of ovarian cancer, as they suppress ovulation, not because of the oestrogen or progestogen they contain. Using birth-control pills for two years reduces your risk by 40 to 50 per cent. Using birth-control pills for five years reduces your risk by 60 to 80 per cent.

Fertility drugs that increase the number of eggs you release during ovulation or increase the number of ovulations you have over a lifetime can increase your risk of ovarian cancer. Again, the blood hormone levels don't create the problem; rather, the physical wear and tear of ovulation is the problem.

Assessing your risks

Ovarian cancer affects one in every 25 women, most of whom are over 50 years of age. This form of cancer is deadly because it usually goes unnoticed until the advanced stages of the disease, so always report suspicious symptoms that are persistent, however vague. Certain factors increase your risks for ovarian cancer:

- A family history of ovarian cancer (mother, sister, or daughter) or breast cancer (mother or sister)
- Using fertility drugs to stimulate your ovaries to release multiple follicles during a single ovulation
- Age over 50
- Never having a pregnancy

Vaginal cancer

Vaginal cancer is rare, with less than 300 women developing this condition in the UK each year. This cancer most commonly affects women aged 50 to 70 years. Although the cause of many vaginal cancers remains unknown, the same types of genital wart virus that cause cervical cancer are probably involved. If a women takes the synthetic oestrogen drug diethylstilboestrol during pregnancy, vaginal cancer may develop in the female offspring. HRT is not known to have any impact on vaginal cancer.

Chapter 14

Revealing the Links between HRT and Other Health Conditions

*I*n Chapters 11–13 we look in detail at the relationships (positive, negative, and neutral) between hormone replacement therapy (HRT) and cardiovascular disease, breast cancer, and other forms of cancer. But, from time to time, you probably read newspaper articles and see reports on the news about a number of other health conditions that may have a link with the use of HRT. We try to set the record straight in this chapter, in which we review a number of conditions you may hear discussed in the same breath as HRT. But, in most instances, research doesn't convincingly show HRT to impact on these conditions one way or the other.

In this chapter we define various conditions, discuss their signs and symptoms, and review how the conditions are linked to HRT. We discuss the symptoms because, regardless of whether they're linked to HRT, these conditions usually affect people over the age of 40, so you may well want to know about them.

Dealing with Deep-Vein Thrombosis and Other Impeding Issues

A *thrombosis* is the medical word for a *blood clot* (a lump of coagulated blood) that forms in a deep vein and impairs the flow of blood. An even more complicated term, which means the same thing, is *phlebothrombosis* (where phlebo- refers to the vein).

How deep do you have to look to find these deep veins? Good question, but contemplating the answer is not as deep as discussing the meaning of life. To find deep veins, you need look no further than the veins in your upper arms, legs, and pelvis, although DVT most commonly occurs in a leg. These veins lie deeper under the skin than surface veins and return more blood to the heart. A clot in one of these veins can cause more complications than a clot in a surface vein, which triggers inflammation called thrombophlebitis.

If a clot forms in one of these deep veins and then breaks off, it can flow to the heart and straight out to the lungs. The process in which a clot forms in a deep vein, then breaks off to travel through the veins is known as *venous thromboembolism*. When a wandering clot (known as an embolus) reaches the lungs, it usually lodges as the veins get smaller and smaller, to cause a blockage that stops blood from reaching the air sacs to pick up oxygen. The blockage is called a *pulmonary embolism – pulmonary* meaning *in the lungs* and *embolism* meaning a *wandering blood clot has lodged.*

A DVT in your upper arm is less likely to cause problems such as a pulmonary embolism than a DVT in your upper thigh or pelvic region. DVTs in the upper part of the leg cause 95 per cent of pulmonary embolisms.

The way in which your blood clots is where hormone replacement therapy enters the explanatory picture. Scientists first discovered the hormone-clot association in women taking birth-control pills. Women who smoke *and* take birth-control pills have a higher incidence of blood clots and *phlebitis* (inflammation of a vein) than other women. A large body of research looking at hormone replacement therapy and blood-clotting conditions, such as DVT and pulmonary embolism, is now available, and growing all the time, with obvious patterns forming.

Recognising the signs

The most troublesome and common cases of DVT occur in the calf and thigh of your leg. We recommend that you know how to recognise a DVT, although keep in mind that only about half of people with a DVT in their leg have symptoms. If you do have symptoms, you may notice some of the following:

- ✔ **Pain or tenderness:** Symptoms may occur in your calf or thigh, sometimes only when standing or walking.

- ✔ **Redness:** Your leg may look red as though you have bumped it.

- ✔ **Swelling:** Your entire leg may swell, or the swelling may affect just a blood vessel, which creates a ridge of swelling that you can feel.

- ✔ **Warmth:** Your leg may feel warm to the touch.

And here's how you can recognise a blood clot in your lung (pulmonary embolism):

- ✔ Chest pain that gets worse with a deep breath
- ✔ Cough that may bring up blood
- ✔ Sudden shortness of breath

Your calf or thigh is the most likely location for a blood clot – at least the first time you get one. Clots like these are likely to cause considerable pain – enough pain that most people call their doctor or go to the hospital. That's a good instinct to follow because these clots need early treatment before they damage nearby tissues or break off and travel toward the lungs.

Sometimes, a leg that has a blood clot can become bluish in colour because the blood is having a hard time getting back to the heart. The blood is blue rather than red because it no longer contains much oxygen. After blood delivers its oxygen to other parts of the body, it returns to the lungs for an oxygen refill.

Determining the role of hormones

Studies in the mid-1990s flip-flopped on the hormone issue. Some research indicated that women on oestrogen therapy are more likely to have blood clots in the legs, *phlebitis* (inflammation of the veins), and *pulmonary embolus* (blood clots in the lung). Other studies showed no clotting-related effects at all. Now that's a lot of help, isn't it?

But a growing body of evidence exists, including the Women's Health Initiative (WHI) study, that shows a correlation between the use of conjugated oestrogen therapy and blood-clotting problems. A variety of studies, including the WHI, found that the risk of DVT or pulmonary embolism doubles in women who use conjugated equine oestrogen. The risk is greatest during the first year of use.

In the UK, the Committee on Safety of Medicines estimates that about 10 in every 1,000 women aged 50–59 years not using HRT develops a venous thromboembolism over five years; this figure rises to 11 per 1,000 (that is, one extra case) in women using oestrogen-only HRT and to 14 per 1,000 women (about 4 extra cases) in women using combined HRT for five years. The risk rises with age, so that 20 in every 1,000 women aged 60–69 years who don't use HRT develop venous thromboembolism over five years; this figure goes up to 24 per 1,000 women (about 4 extra cases) in those using oestrogen-only HRT and to 29 per 1,000 (about 9 extra cases) in those using combined HRT for five years.

Researchers don't know whether tibolone (a synthetic hormone with both oestrogen and progestogen actions) increases the risk of venous thromboembolism.

Major surgery under general anaesthetic significantly increases your risk of DVT due to immobility and due to blood-clotting proteins produced during the healing process. If you are having planned, elective surgery, your doctor is likely to ask you to stop taking HRT four to six weeks before your operation and restart only when you are fully recovered and fully mobile again. If you cannot stop HRT (for example, if you need an unexpected, urgent operation) then your doctor will probably give you a drug (heparin) to thin your blood and recommend that you wear graduated compression stockings.

So, doctors know that HRT increases your risk of a DVT. What they don't really know is why or how. Some researchers believe that *not all forms of oestrogen* have this effect on women. They believe that the *type* of oestrogen (conjugated oestrogen) is responsible for the increase in clotting. Conjugated equine oestrogens, such as those tested by the WHI, are a more potent form of oestrogen than oestrogens found naturally in your body, and may cause unwanted effects. Research in the future may show that hormone therapy using natural oestradiol (which the body uses more easily than conjugated equine oestrogen) won't increase the risk of DVT or pulmonary embolism. Some researchers also question whether it is the conjugated oestrogen or the use of a progestogen that raises the risk of clotting; oestrogen alone doesn't seem to increase the clotting risk as significantly. These researchers suggest that using combined oestrogen and progestogen is more risky.

The hormone-delivery method may also make a difference to your risk of developing clotting problems such as DVT or pulmonary embolism. The WHI study tested only an oral form of oestrogen, and many women receive HRT through a skin-patch, skin gel or nasal spray. Some doctors and researchers suggest that we can't draw conclusions about these other delivery methods based on tests involving an oral form of the hormone. Medical folks know that our bodies process the oestrogen in a patch differently from oestrogen in a pill. Oestrogen given as a pill is processed in the liver before travelling around the body in the bloodstream; oestrogen given via a patch, skin gel, or nasal spray bypasses the liver and is therefore given in a much smaller dose. Chapter 10 provides more information on all the different forms of oestrogen and delivery methods.

So far, the skin-patch, gel and nasal spray delivery methods aren't linked to a higher than normal incidence of blood-clotting problems or phlebitis. However, more research and time are needed to confirm whether non-pill methods of delivering oestradiol are less harmful than conjugated oestrogen pills. In the meantime, carefully consider the risk of DVT and other blood-clotting problems, particularly when using conjugated oestrogen pills in hormone therapy.

Approach hormone use cautiously if you have a condition that predisposes you to DVT, such as a personal or family history of deep-vein thrombosis or pulmonary embolism, severe varicose veins, obesity, trauma, or prolonged bed-rest. Your doctor may decide in these cases that the risks of HRT outweigh the benefits. If you and your doctor decide you can use HRT, then a regimen consisting of the oestradiol form of oestrogen delivered through a patch (with the intra-uterine system (IUS) to protect your endometrium if you have not had a hysterectomy) is probably the safest bet.

Dissecting Diabetes

Diabetes is a huge health problem in the United Kingdom. *Diabetes* is associated with high levels of *glucose* (sugar) in the blood due to the body's inability to process glucose properly.

Insulin is a hormone that acts as a key that lets glucose out of your blood into your muscle and fat cells. When the glucose levels in your blood get relatively high, your pancreas releases insulin to help your cells absorb the sugar in your blood and use it for energy. When the pancreas doesn't produce enough insulin, or your cells can't respond to insulin as normal, then diabetes results.

Two basic reasons explain why some people can't transfer glucose from their blood to their cells:

- ✔ Their body can't make enough insulin.
- ✔ The tissues quit responding to insulin and won't take in glucose.

Two main types of diabetes exist:

- ✔ **Type 1 diabetes:** No one knows what causes type 1 diabetes, but the condition appears to run in families, suggesting that genes are involved. Another trigger factor is also needed, however – possibly a viral illness – that makes the body's immune system destroy insulin-making cells in the pancreas.
- ✔ **Type 2 diabetes:** This form of diabetes is the most common form. Eighty per cent of people with this form of diabetes are overweight. Excess weight in combination with age and lack of exercise is usually what triggers type 2 diabetes.

Recognising the signs

Over 2.2 million people have a diagnosis of diabetes in the United Kingdom, and a similar number are walking around with the disease but are unaware of their condition. If three or four of the following symptoms describe your state of affairs, ask your doctor to check you out as soon as possible:

- Extreme thirst (causing you to drink an unusual amount of fluids)
- Frequent urination (in which you pass unusually large amounts of urine)
- Constant hunger
- Unexpected weight loss
- Fatigue
- Itchy skin or genitals
- Pain or numbness in your extremities
- Slow-healing wounds
- Blurred vision

Determining the role of hormones

The science does not show that hormone replacement therapy (HRT) actually leads to diabetes. Some very small and short-term studies suggest that HRT can slightly increase your blood-glucose levels, but don't worry about it. Most other studies find absolutely no increase in risk of diabetes for women who take HRT. The Women's Health Initiative (WHI) study from 2002 doesn't even mention this side effect, so raising your glucose level isn't a big concern if you're using hormone replacement therapy.

Facing the Facts about Fibromyalgia

Ever heard of this one? Well, nearly 80 per cent of people with fibromyalgia are women, and most of them are over 40 years of age. The laundry list of symptoms may make you say 'You're kidding?' but there's no fibbing about fibromyalgia.

Fibromyalgia is a chronic condition in which you experience widespread muscle and soft-tissue pain, tenderness, and fatigue. You may experience pain in up to 18 specific areas that are aptly named *tender points* or *trigger points* (many of which cluster around your neck).

Fibromyalgia is most common in women between the ages of 30 and 50, but a few women are first diagnosed in their seventies.

Recognising the signs

Fibromyalgia symptoms are very general but intense. They include

- ✔ Stiffness and soreness, especially in the morning
- ✔ Extremely tender places on your body, especially where tendons and muscles meet (on the inside of your elbows and in your hips and knees, for example). Pain in 11 of the 18 tender points is usually the threshold doctors look for in diagnosing this condition
- ✔ Difficulty getting a full night's sleep
- ✔ General fatigue
- ✔ Irritability, mood changes, and depression
- ✔ Problems with eye muscles (your eye may turn inward or close slightly)
- ✔ Numbness, burning, or cold sensations in your hands and feet

Some people with fibromyalgia also experience less common problems with their memory or concentration, have difficulty hearing or can't tolerate some sounds, and suffer migraine headaches.

If you have fibromyalgia, or suspect that you do, you may want to check out *Fibromyalgia For Dummies* by Roland Staud with Christine Adamec (Wiley) in addition to reading the following 'Determining the role of hormones' section.

Determining the role of hormones

Doctors don't understand the cause of fibromyalgia well. Most scientists believe that some type of hormonal imbalance causes the condition, but they don't agree on which hormones are unbalanced. Given the symptoms, researchers are focusing their suspicions on the following areas:

- ✔ Brain chemicals that control mood and can also disrupt the sleep cycle
- ✔ Hormones made in the pituitary gland (which is also found in the brain and is sensitive to oestrogen)
- ✔ Deficiencies in growth hormones

A link to female sex hormones also seems likely because fibromyalgia is most likely to occur:

- ✔ In women approaching menopause or who are passed the menopause
- ✔ In women with a new baby (especially women over 35)
- ✔ A few years after a woman has a tubal ligation (sterilisation) or a hysterectomy

Getting the Goods on Gall Bladder Disease

Your gall bladder is a warehouse for *bile,* a greenish liquid that helps you digest fats. The gall bladder is supposed to take bile from your liver and inject it into the intestines via the bile duct, so it can go to work like a detergent breaking down blobs of dietary fat. When you have too much cholesterol in your bile, the cholesterol hardens, forming crystals inside the gall bladder. The crystals then come together to form *gallstones.*

Recognising the signs

Most people with gallstones don't even know they have them. They experience no symptoms and discover they have stones only when they're tested for another condition such as ulcers or kidney stones. Any pain is usually like a dull ache or cramping. But large or numerous gallstones can cause noticeable pain, vomiting, or nausea. The pain comes on fast and strong and lasts from 30 minutes to several hours. You feel it in your upper abdomen under your ribcage. Sometimes the pain radiates, moving all the way through your lower back or up to your right shoulder. Some people also experience nausea and vomiting or a fever.

If you have a high fever or chills, you may have a blocked or inflamed *bile duct* (pathway to the small intestine). A blocked bile duct can also make your urine dark yellow, your stools light in colour, and your skin to take on a yellow cast. The symptoms often occur at night or after eating – especially if you eat a high-fat meal.

If gallstones cause pain or infections, doctors usually remove your gall bladder, but gallstones themselves are rarely a life-threatening condition.

Determining the role of hormones

Oestrogen has a reputation as a promoter of gallstones. When oestrogen is taken in pill form, the oestrogen is first digested in the liver before entering the bloodstream, and tends to increase levels of LDL cholesterol (the bad stuff) within the bile. Raising the level of cholesterol in the bile can increase the risk of gallstone formation.

Taking oestrogen in patch form instead of taking pills may help to avoid gall bladder issues as using the patch avoids an oestrogen trip through your liver.

Looking at Lupus

Lupus is the short name for a disease called *systemic lupus erythematosus.* Although lupus is fairly rare, more women than men get it – particularly women between the ages of 15 and 45.

Because lupus is a disease of the immune system, it attacks nearly every organ in your body. The immune system normally protects your body from infections. However, with lupus, the immune system starts attacking 'friendly' tissues in your own body. This attack creates havoc, causing tissue damage and illness.

Lupus is a complex disease, and researchers have yet to determine the cause. The likely scenario is that no single cause exists. Instead, a combination of genetic, environmental, and possibly hormonal factors may work together to cause the disease.

The hormone connection is curious. If you look at the population in general, only one in 2,000 people has lupus. But, if you consider only women between the ages of 14 and 45 years old, one in 250 has the disease. This fact leads scientists to conclude that female sex hormones are somehow involved in this disease.

Recognising the signs

Lupus can affect many parts of the body, and often attacks the joints, skin, kidneys, heart, lungs, blood vessels, and brain. Although people with the disease have many different symptoms, some of the most common are:

- Extreme fatigue
- Kidney problems
- Painful, swollen, inflamed joints (arthritis)
- Rashes and inflammation
- Unexplained fever

Many women with lupus initially think that their swollen or stiff joints are simply due to arthritis. In fact, some researchers believe that lupus is related to rheumatoid arthritis. If left untreated, lupus can cause many complications.

Determining the role of hormones

Given that women of childbearing age are at greatest risk of lupus, you may not be surprised that researchers have found an increase in lupus among women taking hormone replacement therapy. Doctors don't understand the specifics, but the correlation between female hormones (including those taken as HRT) and lupus looks suspicious.

One particularly large study shows that women who are taking hormone replacement therapy are twice as likely to develop lupus compared with menopausal women not taking HRT. The longer a woman uses oestrogen, the greater her risk of developing the disease. No one knows the reason for these results.

If you have a family history of lupus, you may want to consider an alternative to HRT for your perimenopausal and menopausal symptoms (check out Chapters 16 and 17 for alternatives).

Monitoring Migraines

Scientists don't know the cause of migraines for certain. About one in eight people in the UK experience migraine, and two out of three people who get migraines are women. Most women who have migraines are between the ages of 20 and 59 and have a family history of migraines.

For years, scientists thought that migraine headaches occur when blood vessels in the brain suddenly constrict (get smaller) and then expand. Now researchers suggest that migraines are linked with inherited abnormalities in certain areas of the brain.

Recognising the signs

Migraine headaches are like everyday headaches, but they're a whole lot worse. Migraines are more intense, throb, often affect only one side of the head, and often cause nausea, vomiting, and sensitivity to light and/or noise. Some people also see *auras*, which are flashing lights or blind spots in their field of vision.

Determining the role of hormones

Many factors can trigger a migraine attack, and fluctuations in oestrogen levels is probably one of them. A sudden drop in oestrogen encourages migraine in women who are predisposed to them. Medical folks don't understand the hormone connection well, particularly in light of the new thoughts on what causes migraines, but the following facts are rather interesting:

- ✔ Two thirds of people with migraine are women.
- ✔ Women who have migraines and are still menstruating generally report them during the part of the cycle when oestrogen levels drop.
- ✔ Women often report that migraines go away during pregnancy.

Many women first suffer migraine headaches during their reproductive years, specifically a day or two before their period or the first day or two of their period when oestrogen levels drop. Other women get migraines around the time they ovulate, when oestrogen levels again drop.

Migraines seem to happen when oestrogen drops, so the fact that many women experience migraines in response to menopause isn't too surprising.

The active form of oestrogen in HRT relieves the symptoms associated with migraines. Women on a cyclical hormone therapy regimen (one in which you stop taking oestrogen for a few days each month) are more likely to have migraines because of rapid drops in oestrogen. Continuous hormone therapy may prevent the headaches.

Chapter 15

Making the Decision about HRT

. . . .

In This Chapter

▶ Recognising a variety of opinions on HRT

▶ Connecting the studies to the headlines

▶ Weighing your options during perimenopause and menopause

. . . .

*T*his chapter helps you decide whether or not hormone replacement therapy (HRT) is right for you. Your decisions about coping with perimenopause and menopause, and whether or not to use HRT are likely to change as your health changes, your priorities shift, and new treatment options are launched. This evaluation process doesn't end with a one-time pronouncement that you follow for the rest of your life. You can (and should!) revisit your alternatives periodically. So, please return to this chapter from time to time over the next few years to get as much out of it as possible.

Outlining Attitudes about HRT

Most women going through the change fall into one of three camps when it comes to hormone replacement therapy (HRT).

   ✔ 'Natural is beautiful. If we are meant to have oestrogen all our lives, why do our ovaries pack in?'

   ✔ 'There's no way I can live a day without my hormones!'

   ✔ 'I gave hormones a go, and they're awful. I prefer to put up with the symptoms.'

Over time, you may move from one camp to another – and then back again. If symptoms interfere with your quality of life during perimenopause, you may decide to take hormones for just a few years to ease the transition into menopause, and then taper off medication as your symptoms decrease.

Updating HRT recommendations

The results from the Women's Health Initiative (WHI) study in 2002 almost put the kibosh on hormone replacement therapy (HRT). The WHI study evaluates the use of a combination oestrogen and progestogen as a means of lowering the risk of cardiovascular disease in women. After several years, the clear answer is that this combination of hormones does *not* lower the risk of cardiovascular disease, but actually increases the risk of breast cancer, heart attacks, strokes, and blood clots. Based on these findings, the US National Institute of Health, the sponsor of the study, stopped the trial several years ahead of schedule.

But the WHI findings are neither surprising nor applicable to all forms of HRT. The study evaluates the use of a specific HRT product (conjugated equine oestrogen plus MPA progestogen). This specific oestrogen product, derived from female horse urine, is one that was already known to have problems. Other major studies from the 1980s and 1990s show that horse-derived oestrogens may produce higher risks of heart disease than the natural oestradiol form of oestrogen.

The specific HRT product in the WHI trial uses MPA (medroxyprogesterone acetate) as the progestogen part of the therapy; this also isn't the best choice. Researchers knew some time ago that MPA causes more blood vessel damage and reverses more of the positive effects of oestrogen than natural progesterone.

In essence, the WHI study simply confirms the information that researchers already know after 20 years worth of research. In fairness, the WHI study is one of the biggest, best organised, and best controlled studies of HRT and its effects on women's health ever conducted. If you want to know how conjugated oestrogen and MPA affect women after menopause, the WHI gives hard facts on the benefits and risks.

This particular hormone combination is not widely prescribed in the UK, however, and the exact doses used are not available. Even so, the study makes doctors wonder if *all* HRT regimens may produce the same results. So far, scientists know that pills have different effects than patches, and that conjugated oestrogen has different effects than oestradiol oestrogen. What they don't know is whether these other HRT regimens have the same health risks as the one tested in the WHI study.

The purpose of HRT is to give you a 'healthy' hormone balance. The 'natural is beautiful' group argues that what's normal at 25 isn't normal at 55, and they're correct. Unfortunately, the low levels of oestrogen that are 'normal' at 55 often result in physical and mental discomfort.

The problem is that your body doesn't produce a substitute for oestrogen when your ovaries quit producing the hormone. When your body stops getting the oestrogen it's used to, it lets you know with messages in the form of hot flushes, memory lapses, vaginal dryness, bone loss, and shifting blood cholesterol levels, all of which are typical of a sustained lack of oestrogen. (We give the low-down on all these symptoms in Part II of this book.)

If your family or personal history includes osteoporosis or colorectal cancer, HRT is often the right choice for you, but keep in mind that other medications can help too. (Check out Chapter 17 for information on treating osteoporosis without hormones.)

Taking HRT does present health risks. Oestrogen may encourage the growth of some breast cancers and may cause problems for you if you have gall bladder or liver disease, blood clots, or undiagnosed vaginal bleeding. So how do you decide? Business people often perform cost–benefit analyses, a rational approach in which you list the benefits (or rewards) and the costs (in this case risks) and make a logical decision. The information in this chapter (and the other HRT-related chapters in this book) helps you perform a cost–benefit analysis.

As with any personal decision, consider your values, lifestyle preferences, and personal prejudices – even those that you recognise are quite illogical. Also, look at your medical history and that of your family. You may eventually face the same medical problems that affect your parents, siblings, or grandparents. This chapter helps you sort through these issues, too.

Weighing the Benefits and Risks of HRT

Most women consider hormone replacement therapy (HRT) only because their symptoms make their lives miserable. Only you can determine whether your quality of life is at risk. (Check out the 'Figuring out just how bad it really is' sidebar to get an objective look at your symptoms.)

Bringing on the benefits

HRT relieves perimenopausal and menopausal symptoms and protects your body against a variety of serious medical conditions. You can find information about these benefits throughout this book (Chapter 10 is a good place to start), but this chapter puts them all together so that you can do a quick side-by-side comparison as you're trying to make your decision. HRT relieves the following:

- Bone deterioration
- Fuzzy thinking
- Hot flushes
- Insomnia and fitful sleep due to hot flushes or night sweats
- Memory lapses
- Vaginal dryness and *atrophy* (thinning and shrinking)

Figuring out just how bad it really is

This quiz is designed to help you decide whether you're experiencing perimenopausal symptoms and, if so, whether they're interfering with your quality of life. The responses are ranked in order from least debilitating to most. The more debilitating, the greater the chance that these symptoms are interfering with your life. The quiz has no target scores – you're the judge.

How often do you experience hot flushes or night sweats?

✔ Never.

✔ Several times a week, but I can deal with it.

✔ Several times a day, and they interfere with my activities.

✔ So often that I'm going nuts.

How often do you experience interrupted sleep or insomnia?

✔ About the same as I have in the past.

✔ Once in a while, but I simply don't sleep as well as I used to.

✔ I wake up a couple of times a night, and I have a hard time getting back to sleep.

✔ I feel like a zombie because I'm awake so much of the night.

Do you feel irritable, anxious, or apprehensive?

✔ No more than usual.

✔ I'm more irritable, anxious, or apprehensive than before.

✔ I sometimes cry at the drop of a hat, and other times I don't want anyone near me.

✔ I'm driving my family and colleagues nuts as I keep flying into a rage.

Are you experiencing vaginal dryness, burning, or itching?

✔ No more than usual.

✔ Intercourse is uncomfortable at times.

✔ My partner and I have cut down on sex as it's painful, and I feel itchy and uncomfortable.

✔ My vagina feels uncomfortable and itchy when doing everyday activities.

Do you experience any other perimenopausal problems?

✔ I experience perimenopausal-like symptoms before my period, but then they go away.

✔ I've noticed my headaches are getting more frequent.

✔ My skin feels prickly, like bugs are crawling on me.

✔ I leak urine when I laugh, exercise, or sneeze.

✔ I seem to leak urine no matter what type of activity I'm doing.

✔ I have frequent memory lapses and have a hard time concentrating.

✔ My heartbeat flutters or pounds rapidly, sometimes when I'm just sitting or resting.

If you experience many of these symptoms but they appear at about the same time each month – before your period – and then go away for a length of time during each menstrual cycle, you probably have premenstrual syndrome (PMS) rather than perimenopausal symptoms.

Some evidence suggests that the mental and emotional symptoms are actually worse during perimenopause than after you're officially menopausal. The wild hormone fluctuations are probably the culprit.

If you're experiencing many of the perimenopausal symptoms described in the 'Figuring out just how bad it really is' sidebar, but they appear at about the same time each month – during the two weeks before your period starts – and then go away for the rest of your menstrual cycle, you probably have premenstrual syndrome rather than perimenopausal symptoms.

Raising the level of oestrogen in your body during the latter 20 to 40 years of your life can protect you against a number of disabling conditions, including the following:

✔ Cardiovascular disease, which includes heart attack (although the connection between oestrogen and cardiovascular disease is not clear cut)

✔ Colon cancer

✔ Elevated LDL ('bad' cholesterol) and *triglyceride* (another bad type of circulating fat) levels

✔ Osteoporosis (weakening of the bones)

Perhaps you're the type of woman who marches through perimenopause, refusing to let those annoying symptoms interfere with your life. You may feel that getting relief from the symptoms just isn't worth the risks that HRT may contribute to other health problems. Or perhaps you barely experience any symptoms.

As you approach menopause, the risks and rewards of HRT may look different to you. The statistics, which we put on paper in the following sections, are fairly dramatic and may help balance the decision scales for you. You may even throw up your hands and say 'Damned if I do, damned if I don't!' What can you do to sort through the decision-making process? Read on. As you read, take into account your family medical history and personal health concerns. And keep in mind that you can always take a fresh look at the situation next month or next year.

Helping your heart stay healthy

Out of a group of 100 women who are 50 years old, 20 of them develop heart disease before their 80th birthday. But, if you put all 100 women on hormones, only 10 develop heart disease before they turn 80. Figure 15-1 provides a graphic representation.

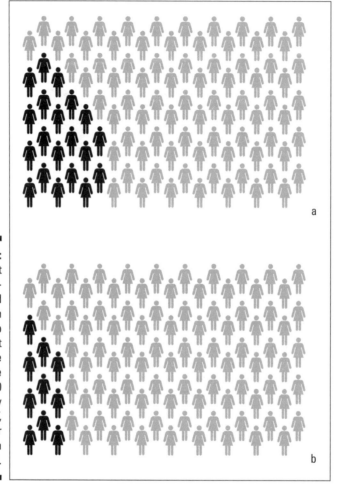

Figure 15-1:
Twenty out
of 100 50-
year-old
women
develop
heart
disease
before
they're 80
(a). If they
all take HRT,
that number
is cut in
half (b).

Pretty impressive, but here's the caveat: During the first and second years of hormone use, your risk of heart disease is actually greater than if you don't take hormones. After the second year, researchers are divided on the benefits of hormone replacement therapy. A large study, the Nurses' Health Study, found the risk of heart disease decreases after the second year of hormone use, and over time, the use of oestrogen cuts the risk of heart disease in half.

The Nurses' Health Study isn't the only study showing that women using hormone replacement therapy have a lower risk of heart disease. So, many people are surprised that the Women's Health Initiative (WHI) study shows that hormone replacement therapy actually increases the risk of heart disease with extended use. Why does the WHI findings differ so radically from prior studies? Is it the specific combination of conjugated equine oestrogens and the medroxyprogesterone acetate (MPA) as progestogen? Doctors aren't certain about the answer to that question yet, but researchers are fast at work to see whether other types of hormones yield the same result.

The WHI results have already caused the authors of this book to head back and re-evaluate the old studies. What do they find during this re-examination? Women with healthy lifestyles (they exercise, don't drink a lot of alcohol, and eat a healthy diet) have less heart disease than other women whether or not they take hormones, so take a good close look at your own diet and lifestyle.

At this point, hormone replacement therapy seems not to be a first line of defence in treating or preventing heart disease or heart attack. And best to avoid HRT if you have a personal history of heart disease or heart attack. The first line of defence against heart disease and heart attack is, as always, a healthy diet, regular exercise, and an overall healthy lifestyle.

Although researchers decided to stop the WHI study early, they didn't put the brakes on due to discovering grave danger to women of dying from a heart attack or heart disease. (Although use of this type of hormone replacement therapy seems to increase the risk of heart attack, it doesn't increase the risk of dying from a heart attack.) Researchers halted the study because of the increase in the risk of breast cancer.

What about other types of cardiovascular disease such as fatty blood (high LDL and triglyceride levels) and *hypertension* (high blood pressure)? Glad you ask. Oestrogen is a mixed bag as far as cholesterol and triglycerides are concerned:

 ✔ Oestrogen lowers LDL levels (by as much as 15 per cent in one study).

 ✔ Some forms of oestrogen raise HDL ('good' cholesterol) levels.

 ✔ Oral oestrogen seems to increase triglycerides (boo!), but the patch tends to lower triglycerides (hurrah!).

The moral of the story is that if you have a problem with blood cholesterol and triglycerides, you need to find the right type of oestrogen to keep them in check.

Oestrogen helps to dilate blood vessels and improve blood flow, both of which are expected to lower your blood pressure. Blood pressure tends to rise with age, however, so ensure that your doctor checks your blood pressure regularly.

High doses of oestrogen seem to increase the risk of stroke slightly in menopausal women. High doses are not too much of a problem as today's HRT regimens use low-dose oestrogen. The Committee on Safety of Medicines estimates that around 3 in every 1,000 women aged 50–59 years not using HRT have a stroke over five years; this figure rises to 5 per 1,000 women (2 extra cases) for those using oestrogen-only HRT. For older women, around 26 in every 1,000 aged 60–69 years not using HRT have a stroke over five years; this figure rises to 32 per 1,000 women (6 extra cases) in those using oestrogen-only HRT.

Lifting the veil on combination HRT and your heart

Now, when you add *progestogen* (synthetic forms of the hormone progesterone) to hormone replacement therapy, everything changes. Progestogens seem to dull the positive effects of oestrogen on your cardiovascular system. HRT containing oestrogen and progestogen:

- ✔ Lowers HDL cholesterol (when taken in pill form).
- ✔ Raises triglycerides (when taken in pill form).

Unfortunately, if you still have your uterus and want to take HRT, the progestogen is vital to protect against endometrial cancer. But a variety of progestogens are available, and patches have less of a negative impact on cholesterol than pills. Before the WHI study, most doctors agreed that HRT may lower your risk of cardiovascular problems. Most doctors now agree that combination HRT is not a good first line of defence against cardiovascular disease.

So, here's the 64-million-dollar question: Is it that conjugated oestrogen and MPA progestogen (the hormone replacement therapy tested in the WHI study) produces more hazardous side effects than other, more natural, forms of hormone replacement therapy (oestradiol and natural progesterone, for example)? Stay tuned for the answer. You can't really take the results of the WHI study and say that all combination hormone replacement therapy regimens create the same hazards to your cardiovascular system. But just so that you know, here's what the WHI study concludes regarding that particular combination of HRT:

- ✔ The risk of stroke doesn't increase during the first year of HRT use, but the risk increases over time – after the first year for about five years (even in healthy women).

✔ Your risk of suffering a heart attack increases while taking HRT, but you're not more likely to *die* of a heart attack while taking HRT compared with women who don't take HRT at all.

Avoiding bone breaks

HRT reduces your risk of osteoporosis and the debilitating results of the disease (check out Figure 15-2). The top figure (a) shows the number of women out of 100 who suffer a hip fracture after the age of 50. The next figure (b) shows the number of hip fractures in women aged 50 or older who take hormone replacement therapy.

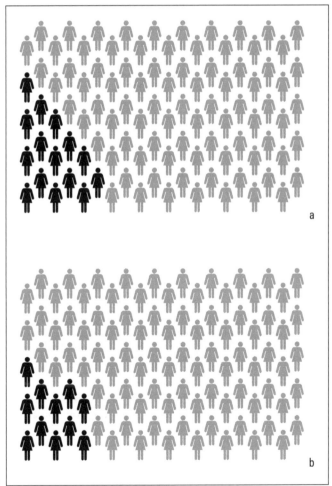

Figure 15-2:
Risk of hip fracture in women aged 50 and older without HRT (a) and with HRT (b).

Most women lose about 3 per cent of bone mass each year after menopause. Postmenopausal women who take HRT regularly for ten years don't lose bone mass; they actually increase their bone mass by about 6 per cent!

Because women on HRT regimens lose less bone (or even build bone) during menopause, they also have a lower incidence of hip fractures. HRT users are about 25 per cent less likely to fracture a hip. That statistic is pretty significant, particularly when you consider how debilitating hip fractures are to women after menopause. (Many women require care for the rest of their life after suffering a broken hip.)

The protective effects of HRT on your bone last only as long as you take hormones. So when you stop – wham! – you begin losing bone mass quickly.

Keeping colon cancer at bay

Here's another one of those 'we don't exactly know why, but it does' benefits of HRT. While you take HRT, you have a slightly lower risk of developing colon cancer. After you discontinue using hormones, the protection gradually disappears.

Regarding the risks

Although hormone replacement therapy is effective at relieving peri-menopause symptoms, and brings some health benefits, like most things in life it also presents some risks. When deciding whether or not to prescribe HRT, doctors only prescribe treatment if they predict that the benefits outweigh the risks. Some of the risks associated with HRT include the following:

- ✔ **HRT increases your risk of endometrial cancer if you take oestrogen without also taking progesterone.** Today, doctors no longer prescribe oestrogen without balancing it with progesterone, so this isn't much of a problem anymore. Unless you have had a hysterectomy, your doctor won't prescribe oestrogen alone (see Chapter 13 for more on endometrial cancer).

- ✔ **HRT increases your risk of gall bladder problems.** Although HRT increases your risk of gallstones (particularly when taken in pill form for more than five years), researchers don't know why the increase in risk occurs (we talk about gallstones in Chapter 14). The risk is lower if you use a patch instead of a pill.

- **HRT may increase your risk of breast cancer.** Some breast cancers, but not all breast cancers, depend on oestrogen to grow. Because HRT raises oestrogen levels, taking it may encourage oestrogen-related breast cancer. The evidence is stacking up on the breast cancer issue – find the low-down in Chapter 12.

- **HRT may increase your risk of deep-vein blood clots.** If you experienced clotting during a pregnancy or while using birth-control pills, you may have a problem with HRT as well, particularly if you smoke. In Chapter 14 we talk about the relationship between clots and HRT.

- **HRT may increase your risk of heart attack and coronary heart disease.** The scales are starting to tip in the direction that HRT may actually increase your risk of heart problems rather than lowering it. The jury is still out: The increased risk is less true of HRT that uses skin-patches/gel as the method of delivery, and oestradiol as the oestrogen, as opposed to other forms of HRT delivery. We weigh up the heart risks and benefits of HRT in Chapter 11.

Having trouble deciding whether you're at risk for osteoporosis, cardiovascular disease, or breast cancer? We present three little quizzes to help you look objectively at your risk factors. The lists in Figures 15-3, 15-4, and 15-5 are a simple first step to assessing your risks – high, medium or low. You can't predict your chances of getting a particular disease from your answers, but the more statements you agree with, the greater your risk for that condition.

Risk is not the same as *certainty*. We all know people who smoke and drink and live long lives, and others who live healthily and exercise and yet die of a heart attack well before their time. But, in between these unlikely extremes, you can evaluate your risk factors and take steps to improve your chances of preventing disease.

Many women choose to weigh their risk of osteoporosis against their risk of breast cancer as HRT helps to protect you from osteoporosis but may raise your risk for breast cancer.

If you are at great risk of osteoporosis but have few risk factors for breast cancer, you may feel warm and fuzzy towards HRT. If you're at great risk for breast cancer, you may want to consider other alternatives for protecting your bones: In Chapters 16–19 we give you great ideas about alternatives.

Some of the risk factors for osteoporosis and breast cancer are things you can control through modifying your lifestyle, eating preferences, or other behaviours. Making simple changes can lower these risks immediately.

Osteoporosis Risk Sheet

1. My mother and/or sister has osteoporosis.
2. I am 'small-boned'.
3. I am white or Asian.
4. I am older than 65 years of age.
5. I breast fed for at least three months.
6. I have lost at least an inch in height.
7. I have taken cortisone or corticosteroids for over five years.
8. My periods stopped before I was 40.
9. My ovaries were removed before I was 40.
10. I get less than 1,200 mg of calcium each day.
11. I exercise for less than one and a half hours a week.
12. I smoke.
13. I was anorexic for a period in my life.
14. I drink three or more cups of coffee a day (or the equivalent amount
    of caffeine as found in colas, chocolate, and so on).

**You are in a higher risk category for osteoporosis if you agree with
questions 1–4.**

Figure 15-3:
Evaluating
your risk
for osteo-
porosis.

Heart Disease Risk Sheet

1. My mother had a heart attack before she was 65 years old/my dad had
   a heart attack before he was 55 years old.
2. I have had a heart attack.
3. I have hypertension (high blood pressure).
4. My HDL cholesterol is less than 50.
5. My cholesterol to HDL ratio is over 3.0.
6. My triglycerides are over 120.
7. I have diabetes.
8. I have chest pain (angina) or heart flutters (fibrillation) on occasion.
9. I typically eat more than 50 grams of fat a day.
10. I smoke.
11. I'm overweight.
12. I exercise less than three times a week or for less than an hour and a half a week.

Figure 15-4:
Evaluating
your risk
for heart
disease.

> ### Breast Cancer Risk Sheet
>
> 1. I have had breast cancer.
> 2. My mother or sister has had breast cancer.
> 3. My grandmothers had breast cancer.
> 4. There is colon, endometrial, ovarian, or cervical cancer in my family.
> 5. I gave birth to my first child after age 35.
> 6. I am over 35 and have never had a baby.
> 7. I have at least three alcoholic drinks a week.
>
> **Agreeing with the first three statements puts you in a fairly high risk category.**

Figure 15-5:
Evaluating your risk for breast cancer.

Some studies indicate that HRT slightly increases your risk of breast cancer, but other studies show no effect whatsoever. If you're worried about your risk of breast cancer, take an objective look at your personal risk factors for the disease.

Summing Up the Studies

If you've read the rest of this chapter, you've digested a lot of information, and your plate is probably still full. Here's a little synopsis to help you separate your peas from your potatoes, regroup, re-energise, and re-weigh the risks and benefits associated with hormone replacement therapy.

The best-studied type of HRT is the regimen in which you take a daily pill that contains both conjugated equine oestrogen and MPA progestogen, but this blend is not common in the UK. Studies of other regimens are more varied in terms of the size of their study group and the types of HRT they investigate. So the results below show a heavy bias towards the benefits and risks of combination therapy using conjugated oestrogen and MPA progestogen. For more information on all the different types of therapies and hormones, check out Chapter 10. For now, Tables 15-1 and 15-2 provide a summary of the short- and long-term benefits and risks of HRT.

Studying the studies: What you need to know before you panic over news stories

Conflicting reports on the risks and benefits of HRT make the decision about taking HRT really confusing. Magazines, newspapers, and talking heads on TV constantly present you with new studies proving that everything you read in the past is wrong. The reports cut both ways. One week someone says the risks of HRT are blown way out of proportion. The next week you read that HRT does absolutely nothing to help menopausal women. (See the 'Updating HRT recommendations' sidebar earlier in this chapter.)

One reason opinions swing so far in each direction is nothing whatsoever to do with HRT itself but everything to do with how the studies are conducted. Without getting too complicated, experts basically conduct three types of studies: descriptive, observational, and controlled trials.

Descriptive studies simply describe what happens to patients or groups of people. For example, one doctor may report that all her patients who experience hot flushes have blue eyes. From this information, you can't really say that blue eyes cause hot flushes, but such a report is interesting to experts studying hot flushes (or experts studying people with blue eyes).

Observational studies observe people in the settings of their everyday lives. Researchers interview study participants over an extended period of time about their lifestyles, medical histories, existing medical conditions, and medications. A good thing about observational studies is that you can find a good-sized group of people who are taking a medication or participating in a therapy over a long period of time. The disadvantage is that no real *control* is in place. Participants do whatever they want and don't have to limit themselves to one particular therapy. You can detect patterns, but you can only speculate about what causes those patterns.

Controlled trials participants are generally in two groups – one that uses the therapy of interest and a *control group* that takes a *placebo* (form of therapy that outwardly resembles the therapy under test but provides no medicinal or curative properties) or nothing at all. In these kinds of studies, researchers can determine the cause if a change occurs. The best controlled trials are *randomised,* meaning that researchers randomly assign people to a therapy group. Comparisons of the groups are objective, without the possibility that the person sorting the participants may accidentally put all the sick people in one group and all the healthy people in the other, for example.

Basically, each type of study has merits and drawbacks. Descriptive and observational studies can shed light on patterns of disease or medical conditions, but they can't demonstrate the exact *cause* of a particular effect. You can show that some kind of link exists between certain factors and a particular disease or condition, but you can't really describe the details of the link. Controlled studies are designed to determine causes. That doesn't mean that controlled trials are the only valuable studies, although many experts insist that controlled, randomised trials are the only way to go when making medical recommendations.

The next time you see an alarming headline in your favourite magazine or newspaper that casts doubt on everything you've ever read about menopause or HRT, read the details. Make sure that the conclusions drawn from the study (and the resulting claims) don't reach further than the study method permits. But also make sure that researchers and writers aren't throwing the baby out with the bath water – dismissing studies simply because they aren't randomised, controlled trials.

Table 15-1	Just the Facts, Part I: HRT Benefits during Use
Short-Term Use (Less Than 5 Years)	*Long-Term Use (5 Years or More)*
Improves mental skills (verbal memory and reasoning)	Increases bone density
Improves sense of well-being	Reduction of hip fractures
Decrease in sleep interruption	Reduction of spinal fractures
Decrease in *urogenital atrophy* (atrophy of the vagina and urinary tract)	Reduction of colon cancer
Decrease in mood swings	Decrease in dementia
Decrease in hot flushes	

Table 15-2	Just the Facts, Part II: HRT Risks during Use
Short-Term Use (Less Than 5 Years)	*Long- Term Use (5 Years or More)*
Possible increase in breast cancer	Increase in breast cancer
Increase in gall bladder disease	Significant increase in gall bladder disease
Increase in heart attack	Slight increase in heart attack
Slight increase in stroke	Slight increase in stroke
Significant increase in deep-vein clots	Increase in deep-vein clots

Presenting the Options for Perimenopause

In the following sections we describe several ways that women deal with perimenopausal symptoms. You may want to mix and match the various options. For example, although we list diet, exercise, herbal solutions, and HRT in separate sections, adopting better eating and exercise habits probably enhances the positive aspects of herbs and HRT.

Option 1: The lifestyle solution

If you're perimenopausal and your symptoms annoy you but rarely interfere with your life, you may want to make lifestyle changes to alleviate them. (Munch through Chapters 18 and 19 to help renew your commitment to keeping your body fit and healthy in this new season of your life.) Many women find that some of the symptoms of perimenopause fade with a renewed focus on getting or staying fit.

Some of the anxiety and irritability you're experiencing probably stems from feeling out of control about the changes going on with your body. Adding a few pounds in weight per year and losing muscle tone isn't unusual for perimenopausal women, but these things are not due to changes in your hormones. As people move into their forties and fifties, they often devote less time to their personal needs than they devote to the demands of their families and careers. A healthy diet and exercise plan can put you in control of your body and improve your state of mind.

Regular physical activity improves mental functions such as memory, concentration, self-confidence, and self-esteem. Exercise also reduces stress, which can trigger hot flushes, interrupted sleep, and irritability. But the effects of exercise are not all mental. Only about 1 in 20 women who exercise regularly report experiencing hot flushes, compared to 1 out of 4 less-active women.

Eating a healthy diet, as we describe in Chapter 18, boosts your immune system, helps maintain bone density, and keeps your blood lean, so you lower your risk of cardiovascular disease and reverse some of the effects of the low oestrogen levels that define menopause.

Incorporating soy into your diet helps lower your cholesterol, boosts your immune system, and prevents hot flushes, and it may lower your risk of breast cancer, too. (Check out Chapter 16 for more on soy.)

Option 2: The complementary solution

For most women, perimenopausal symptoms are not life-threatening, and so using drugs and hormones to relieve symptoms may seem like using a shotgun to kill mosquitoes.

You may want to consider non-HRT alternatives to alleviate your symptoms. These alternatives are as diverse as herbs, relaxation techniques, and vaginal lubricants. Herbs of interest for relieving perimenopausal symptoms include black cohosh, soy, dong quai, and ginseng. In Chapter 16 we look at herbal solutions in more detail.

Stress often triggers hot flushes and anxiety or irritability, so now is a great time to practise relaxation techniques regularly. Don't worry: You don't need to visit Nepal to find a guru. Just take a few minutes each day to do an activity you enjoy, practise breathing techniques, and give someone a hug. *Biofeedback techniques* (psychological therapy in which you use your mind to control certain body functions) can help you to take charge of your breathing and heart rate and lessen your reaction to stressful events or situations. Find out what works for you to reduce the stress in your life – perhaps you should take up yoga, walking, music, or a weekly massage. In Chapter 16 we explore alternative options more fully.

Option 3: The HRT solution

If your symptoms are interfering with your quality of life, HRT is a possible answer – even if you aren't wild about taking medication. HRT relieves hot flushes because oestrogen helps regulate body temperature. In addition, oestrogen improves sleep and lowers anxiety as it increases the production and extends the action of *serotonin* (a brain chemical that regulates moods and activity level). Serotonin boosts concentration, improves pain tolerance, enhances memory, and regulates adrenaline so that you avoid heart palpitations. Progesterone is only added to the HRT regimen to reduce the risk of endometrial cancer that oestrogen-only HRT presents.

Many women choose to take HRT to get rid of their annoying perimenopausal symptoms and enjoy added protection for their bones.

If you decide that HRT is for you, you still have the option of not using the therapy later on. After a few years, perimenopausal symptoms subside (they don't last forever), and doctors usually recommend that you limit your use of HRT to perimenopause.

The HRT option is almost a requirement for women whose ovaries are removed before menopause. Often HRT is prescribed before or immediately after such surgery. Removal of your ovaries is quite a shock to your body because hormone production abruptly ceases. HRT can help absorb the shock as it replaces the hormones and smoothes things over so you don't experience intense menopausal symptoms, bone loss, or changes in your blood cholesterol.

Remember that many types of oestrogen and progesterone are available in many different combinations. Some combinations may make you feel worse; others may make you feel better. If you're feeling worse, don't simply continue with the regimen or just give up – go back to your doctor and discuss the situation. While you're working the kinks out of your HRT programme, monitor your symptoms and any adverse reactions and write them down. Having notes with you when you visit your doctor can help make the meeting more productive. You can accurately describe your symptoms and reactions to your doctor, and the two of you can come up with a treatment plan that works for you. If you're not comfortable with your doctor, find a medical advisor with whom you can work.

You and your doctor may have to try a couple of different formulas to find the correct therapy for you. Think of a hospital gown: One size doesn't fit everyone.

Quitting HRT

If you're taking HRT when you hit menopause, then this is a good time to re-evaluate your situation and consider the benefits you want to gain from hormone replacement therapy. As you reconsider your decision, talk to your doctor. *Do not* simply stop taking HRT. If you choose to quit taking HRT, your doctor is the person in the best position to guide you. You need to consider what you want to do about preventing health problems associated with sustained, low levels of oestrogen.

Differences exist between the benefits and risks of long-term HRT use and short-term HRT use (see Tables 15-1 and 15-2 for a summary). The risks you're most worried about are often not a problem (or as big a problem) if you're taking HRT for just a short while – just long enough to get you through the perimenopausal symptoms. According to the Women's Health Initiative study, preventing cardiovascular disease is no longer a good reason to begin HRT. To reduce heart disease and cardiovascular risks, improve your diet, get more exercise, and quit smoking. These methods are absolutely safe and proven to reduce your risk of cardiovascular problems, including heart attack and stroke.

Finding Your Comfort Zone

This chapter takes a look at risk factors for various medical conditions that are associated with oestrogen or the lack of it. But you can't make a decision about HRT without considering your lifestyle and your personal preferences. Some women are frightened about taking yet another medication; others fear having a heart attack. Some women make a concerted effort to improve their health by committing to more exercise and a healthier diet; others are dedicated couch potatoes. Some women have families who support new endeavours; other women's families ridicule change. The following sections help you assess some of these touchy-feely personal values to see whether you're likely to protect your health more successfully using diet, exercise, and non-HRT alternatives or whether HRT presents you with the best chance for success. Consider these factors as a piece of your HRT decision-making puzzle.

Twelve signs that HRT isn't for you

To get an HRT programme working for you, you have to communicate well with your doctor and share a sense of trust with him or her. If you aren't in that frame of mind, you may not have success with your HRT programme. And, if you're the type of woman who is wary of traditional medicine, pharmaceuticals, and synthetic drugs, you may want try a few of the alternatives to HRT. You can always re-evaluate your condition and your comfort zone in the future.

Read the following statements and see whether you agree with them. If you're in agreement with a lot of these statements, you may want to try HRT alternatives, including a healthy diet, exercise, herbal alternatives, and other preventative treatments.

1. I've had breast cancer.

2. My mother, sister, or daughter has had breast cancer.

3. I have coronary heart disease.

4. I don't have, or I can live with, hot flushes, interrupted sleep, or other symptoms due to hormonal changes.

5. I have a history of unexplained blood clots, deep-vein thrombosis, or blood clots in my lungs (*pulmonary embolism*).

6. I don't like taking medication, and I believe that herbs can do a better job than drugs.

7. I typically eat a healthy diet that includes at least five servings of fruits and vegetables a day.

8. I exercise regularly, and I'm successful at maintaining my target weight.

9. I think that doctors and pharmaceutical companies are just out to make money from women going through menopause.

10. I haven't gone to a doctor in years and don't plan on starting now.

11. My mother said she never had any problems going through menopause without hormones, and I don't think that I will either.

12. I have very few risk factors for osteoporosis or cardiovascular disease.

Top ten signs that you're a good candidate for HRT

No one wants to take medicine just to take it. Women who take HRT during menopause are concerned about preventing disease or eliminating discomfort. To find a successful HRT regimen, you must have confidence in your doctor and understand why you're making this decision, because you may have to experiment for a while to find the right hormone regimen. If you find yourself agreeing with some of these statements, you may want to consider HRT.

1. I have a lot of osteoporosis in my family.

2. My mother or grandmother broke her hip.

3. I'm miserable with these hot flushes and mood swings, and my colleagues and family wish they could send me to the moon.

4. I've taken HRT for a year now and haven't had any trouble.

5. I'm a junk-food junkie and could never survive on rabbit food like vegetables and fruit to stay fit.

6. My sex life is a huge problem as I'm not in the mood for it and intercourse is painful.

7. I don't have a huge number of risk factors for osteoporosis, but I've read the statistics, and I think that I'm at greater risk for that than breast cancer.

8. It seems like a lot of HRT options exist, so I shouldn't have a problem sticking to a schedule.

9. I'm not big on herbal remedies to prevent or treat serious diseases.

10. I have a good rapport with my doctor, and I'd like to give HRT a try to help prevent disease.

If you still have concerns or questions, talk to your doctor. Don't simply stop a therapy that you're taking. Your doctor can help you interpret the information you read about a study. Don't base your decision about HRT – or any medication, for that matter – on TV programmes and newspaper articles.

Chapter 16

Taking an Alternative Route: Non-Hormone Therapies

. . . .

In This Chapter

▶ Seasoning your therapy with herbs

▶ Healing yourself with acupuncture

▶ Subduing your symptoms with biofeedback and yoga

▶ Soothing away your cares with lubricants

. . . .

*A*t least 40 per cent of perimenopausal and menopausal women in the United Kingdom use some form of *non-conventional therapy* (medical therapies not commonly used or previously accepted in conventional Western medicine) to treat their symptoms, alongside or instead of hormone replacement therapy (HRT).

If all you want is to eliminate the annoying symptoms of perimenopause, then complementary approaches are probably your best bet, as they generally have fewer complications and risks compared with hormone therapies. But staying healthy during perimenopause and menopause also requires the prevention of more serious health issues that begin when your body starts producing lower levels of oestrogen – you are probably going to need conventional medicines too at times.

Strictly speaking, non-conventional therapies are referred to as *complementary* if you use them in addition to conventional medicine, and *alternative* if you use them in place of conventional medicine. For example, many women who take HRT also use biofeedback to further reduce stress and anxiety. In this case, biofeedback is considered to be a complementary treatment. (For more on biofeedback, see 'Tuning in to biofeedback' later in this chapter.) An example of an alternative therapy is using the herb black cohosh (which we describe later in the section 'Getting the scoop on individual herbs') instead of hormones to relieve perimenopausal symptoms.

Probably the best way to approach non-conventional therapies is to use them together with conventional medicine so that you get the best of both worlds. In fact, the term 'complementary medicine' is so much better than 'alternative therapies' – as it implies a mutual benefit – that we use the term throughout the rest of this book. The term also reflects the fact that therapies that started out as non-conventional and alternative are now increasingly incorporated into conventional medicine after years of research and success in treatment.

If you're using or considering using complementary medicine, always tell your doctor. If a complementary treatment works for you, your doctor may research the area more thoroughly and suggest the approach to other patients. The main reason to keep your doctor informed, however, is that herbal remedies and food supplements are medicines – they can alter your body functions just as much as drugs from a pharmacy do. (For example, some herbs used to treat menopausal symptoms interfere with anaesthesia during a surgical procedure.) Treat non-conventional approaches as seriously as you treat other medications.

Check out this chapter for interactions and other potential problems before using the most effective non-traditional approaches – herbal remedies, mind–body therapies, biofeedback, and acupuncture.

Ploughing through the Pros and Cons of Herbs

Interest in complementary medicine is growing. Some women enjoy taking a more holistic approach to their lives, including the menopause, while others choose to avoid at least some forms of conventional medicine and hormone therapy for personal reasons – perhaps because someone you know has had a bad experience with a particular therapy. In this section we look at why some doctors are concerned about herbal therapies, and how herbal therapies are getting safer.

Considering the concerns of conventional medicine

Conventional medicine's biggest complaint about herbal complementary therapies concerns the perceived lack of scientific studies surrounding the plants. Some herbs are studied in controlled experiments, but many are not, so researchers aren't always sure whether they work any better than a sugar pill. The placebo effect is a powerful thing, however, and if something works for you, that's great.

Any company that wants to market and sell a herb or plant therapy over the counter as a *medicine* in the United Kingdom must go through an official registration process under European Union legislation known as the Traditional Herbal Medicines Directive. These products have a THR (Traditional Herbal Registration) number on the product labels, meet specific standards of safety and quality, and include an information leaflet to ensure safe use. Previously, a company making medicinal claims about a herb product had to show effectiveness and safety of the product through the same product licensing process as pharmaceutical drugs (these have a PL – Product Licence – number on the label). Herbs that, despite medicinal uses, are accepted as foods (for example, garlic) are sold as food supplements. These do not have to prove effectiveness or safety but on the rare occasion that a product is deemed unsafe it is rapidly recalled under the same process that unsafe foods are withdrawn. Most herbal medicines reach the public as unlicensed herbal remedies, however, which are made up and supplied directly by herbal practitioners. These herbal remedies do not have to meet specific standards of safety or quality, and standards vary widely.

Some herbs are just as dangerous and toxic as drugs. Herbs can interact with other medications that you take and can produce toxic effects if taken in large quantities. Because most herbs aren't tested in recognised studies, warnings about side effects are often sketchy, anecdotal, and not based on clinical trials. Chemicals that are toxic are sometimes included within herbal supplements. (See 'Avoiding Problems with Plants' later in this chapter for more info). The Web site of the Medicines and Healthcare products Regulatory Agency (MHRA) has a section dedicated to Herbal Safety News (www.mhra.gov.uk) that includes information on current safety issues, prohibited and restricted herbal ingredients, side effects and interactions with other medicines.

Conventional medicine's other complaint concerns testing for proper doses of herbs. Many herbs are sold without thorough tests of the effects of taking too large a dose or taking the recommended dose for a long time.

When labels mention *recommended doses,* the definition of that term is often unclear. Who exactly is that dose recommended for – a person who weighs 68 kilograms (10 stone 10 pounds) or a person who weighs 120 kilograms (18 stone 12 pounds)? Should you take more of the supplement if your symptoms are more severe and less if your symptoms are less severe? Is there an upper threshold at which the herb becomes toxic or a lower threshold at which the herb is ineffective? Does the herb interfere with other drugs that you take?

You may have no means of measuring the exact quantity provided in a dose, unless the product is standardised to contain a known quantity. Where possible, always select a supplement whose label states that the product is standardised.

The amount of active ingredient found in each plant varies depending on its genetic background, the soil in which the plant is grown, the time of year, and methods of cultivation. As the quality of different batches of raw material varies significantly, standardisation provides consistency. Standardisation ensures that each batch you buy contains the same amount of one or more active ingredients and provides the same benefit. To achieve this standardisation, the manufacturer concentrates the herbal preparation so that the correct level of ingredient is present. This way, tablets or capsules made from different batches of herb always contain the same, known amount of the medicinal ingredient. One part of a standardised extract is often prepared from as much as 50 parts of dried leaves or more. In contrast, non-standardised products may contain little, if any, active components. Standardised remedies are more likely to have good quality, randomised, double-blind, placebo-controlled trials to support their benefits.

Growing safety into herbal therapy

Before you pick a bottle of herbs off the shelf and incorporate herbal therapies into your life, talk to a qualified herbalist. An experienced, qualified herbalist can suggest the right herbal therapies for you – which is a great alternative to playing the eeny-meeny-miney-mo game at the health food store. A herbalist can help you find herbs that work well together and avoid combinations that have unwanted side effects, helping you to put together your shopping list to make sure that your therapy is as safe and effective as possible.

To find a herbalist, consult a national herbalist organisation (we list some in Appendix B). Most of these professional organisations have codes of ethics to which members must adhere and certification programmes for their members. When looking for a herbalist, take the same investigative steps that you would when looking for a new doctor – ask friends for recommendations and find out about the herbalist's training, practices, philosophy, and experience.

Research into the safety and effectiveness of herbs is much more advanced in Germany than in North America and the United Kingdom. Germany has relatively strict guidelines for regulating herbal supplements, and herbal therapies that meet German standards are more reliable in terms of labelling, the contents, and the amount of active ingredients contained in each dose. These benefits should start to filter through to the UK, thanks to the EU Traditional Herbal Medicines Directive, but for now try to buy herbs that have been certified in Germany.

German health authorities use the guideline of *reasonable certainty,* which means that they consider the experiences of general practitioners – not just clinical trials – in evaluating a plant drug. *The Complete German Commission E Monographs: Therapeutic Guide to Herbal Medicines* (by Mark Blumenthal, published by Integrative Medicine Communications) is an English translation of the German 'safe herb' list (the Commission E report). For more information on herbs, you can also check out *Herbal Remedies For Dummies* by Christopher Hobbs (Wiley).

Relieving Your Symptoms with Plants

Herbal treatments for your mental, emotional, and physical symptoms associated with perimenopause and menopause abound. A lot of these herbal treatments also relieve similar premenstrual symptoms. Herbalists use a number of botanical therapies that are mild, effective, and reliable. Some therapies are tested in clinical trials; others are proven helpful through years of use.

Cataloguing herbal therapies by symptom

If you're wondering what herbal therapy can do for you, here are some of the symptoms that perimenopausal and menopausal women use herbs to relieve and the herbs that are effective in relieving the symptoms:

- **Depression and anxiety:** *Angelica sinensis, Eleutherococcus senticosus, Ginkgo biloba, Glycyrrhiza glabra, Hypericum perforatum, Leonorus cardiaca, Panax ginseng, Verbena hastate, Withania somnifera*

- **Heart palpitations:** *Cimicifuga racemosa, Crataegus oxyacanth, Leonorus cardiaca*

- **Heavy bleeding:** *Achillea millefolium, Alchemilla vulgaris, Capsella bursa-pastoris, Myrica cerifera*

- **Hot flushes and night sweats:** *Actea racemosa, Leonorus cardiaca, Panax ginseng, Salvia officinalis*

- **Insomnia:** *Eleutherococcus senticosus, Glycyrrhiza glabra, Lavendula officinalis, Leonorus cardiac, Passiflora incarnata, Piper methysticum, Scutellaria lateriflora, Valeriana officinalis, Withania somnifera,*

- **Memory problems:** *Bacopa moniera, Paeonia lactiflora, Panax ginseng, Gingko biloba, Rosmarinus officinalis*

- **Vaginal dryness:** *Actaea racemosa, Calendula officinalis, Glycyrrhiza glabra, Panax quinquefolium, Trifolium pratense*

Women in Europe and Asia have used herbs for years to treat the symptoms of perimenopause and menopause. We don't give doses here, however, for a couple of reasons:

- ✔ The quantity of active ingredients varies from brand to brand.
- ✔ You should always seek help from a qualified herbalist before taking herbs.

Herbs are natural, but natural doesn't mean they don't cause side effects. The poison strychnine is natural, too!

Getting the scoop on individual herbs

Many of the herbs used to treat perimenopausal and menopausal symptoms are phytooestrogens (*phyto* means plant, and you know what oestrogen is). *Phytooestrogens* are plant oestrogens – natural sources of oestrogen that act as weak oestrogens and seem to produce oestrogen-effects in menopausal women. In other words, they reduce perimenopausal and menopausal symptoms.

If you take phytooestrogens without a progestogen, you may be at higher risk for endometrial cancer. Phytooestrogens are natural, but they're still mild forms of oestrogen and cause your uterine lining to continue to thicken. If you use phytooestrogens, tell your doctor. He or she can monitor your bleeding and perform tests or recommend therapy as needed. (For more information on unopposed oestrogen therapy, see Chapter 10.)

Tell your doctor if you're taking any of the herbs that we describe here. Some of these herbs interfere with the effectiveness of other medicines. They're considered medicines as in when your doctor asks you, 'What medicines are you taking?'

The following herbs are among the most commonly used by medical herbalists to treat symptoms associated with the menopause.

Ashwagandha (Withania somnifera)

Much like ginseng, eleuthero, and liquorice, ashwagandha is said to reduce stress and depression and aid sleep with long-term use.

Black cohosh (Actaea racemosa syn, Cimicifuga racemosa)

Women have used black cohosh for hundreds, maybe thousands, of years. (Early Native Americans used black cohosh, and other folk medicines made use of it.) Today black cohosh is one of the more commonly used herbs in the battle against perimenopausal symptoms because it relieves hot flushes, vaginal atrophy, tension, elevated blood pressure, restless sleep, and stress. Many of these actions are due to direct effects on the brain rather than through phytooestrogens, however.

Again, black cohosh is a phytooestrogen, so talk to your doctor before using it if you have breast cancer or if you plan on using it for more than three or four months.

If you're going to give black cohosh a go, the German recommendation is to use it for six months or less (to avoid thickening of your endometrium).

Dong Quai (Angelica sinensis)

Also known as *tang gui,* this herb has a history of hundreds of years use in traditional Chinese medicine to 'strengthen the blood'. Dong quai has a blood-thinning action similar to warfarin, so don't use it if you have blood clotting problems. It also seems to eliminate hot flushes.

Dong quai reduces blood clotting, so if you're having surgery let your doctor know beforehand that you're using this herb. You should stop using it two weeks before surgery. Also, don't use dong quai if you have unexplained vaginal bleeding. While using this herb, try to avoid aspirin and other drugs that thin your blood.

Ginkgo (Gingko biloba)

This herb helps to improve your memory and feelings of wellbeing, and one study of 200 women shows that it increases sexual desire. Bring it on!

But don't use it with abandon. Ginkgo also reduces blood clotting (it thins your blood), so always let your doctor know that you're using this herb. If you're undergoing an operation, quit taking ginkgo at least two weeks before surgery. And don't take it if you're taking other blood thinners such as the drug, warfarin, or the herb dong quai.

Ginseng (Panax ginseng, Panax quinquefolium)

People all over the world consume ginseng to increase vitality, improve memory, relieve anxiety, and kick-start low libido. Historically, menopausal women have used ginseng to relieve depression, fatigue, memory lapses, and low libido. It doesn't seem to raise your oestrogen levels or cause your endometrium to thicken as some of the phytooestrogens tend to do.

Take care about using ginseng if you're taking other types of medication for depression or anxiety. Ginseng has been known to cause mania when combined with certain antidepressant medications.

Motherwort (Leonorus cardiaca)

Chinese people have used motherwort for a very long time. Western herbalists make use of it to treat menopausal anxiety, insomnia, heart palpitations, and vaginal atrophy.

Peony (Paeonia lactiflora)

Peony helps to dilate the blood vessels so that blood flows more smoothly through your cardiovascular system. Some people claim that it also improves your mental focus and reduces mental lapses.

Red clover (Trifolium pratense)

Menopausal women often find that this herb, historically used to treat skin and breathing problems, relieves vaginal dryness and lowers their LDL ('bad' cholesterol) levels while increasing their HDL ('good' cholesterol) levels. Red clover contains *isoflavones* (the chemicals that make phytooestrogens work like oestrogen), so it acts as a mild oestrogen.

As with all phytooestrogens, don't use red clover if you have breast cancer.

Sage (Salvia officinalis)

Sage leaf is said to relieve hot flushes, but the claim isn't widely researched.

St John's wort (Hypericum perforatum)

The popularity of St John's wort for treating depression has grown tremendously in recent years. Use of this herb dates back to the Middle Ages. During perimenopause and menopause, women use it to treat mild depression. Although a lot of published reports show that St John's wort is effective, scientists still don't know how it works.

This herb can sensitise the skin so that exposure to sunlight produces a rash in some people. Wear sunscreen and avoid undue sun exposure when using it. If a rash develops, seek medical advice. It also interferes with a variety of other medications, so, as with any herb, tell your doctor that you're taking it.

Soy

Soy is a plant oestrogen (phytooestrogen), so it has the same pros and cons as other phytooestrogens. Soy has been reported to relieve hot flushes, interrupted sleep, anxiety, and other perimenopausal symptoms. However, too much soy has the same effect as unopposed oestrogen (unfettered thickening of the uterine lining).

Although many advertisements for soy products point to the health of women in Japan and China as evidence that they work, women in these cultures start eating soy early in life, and they eat mostly fermented-soy products, such as *miso* (soybean paste) and *tempeh* (a cheese-like soybean food), rather than soy-protein drinks and milk. But studies show that soy can clean up your blood by reducing your total cholesterol, LDL cholesterol (the 'bad' cholesterol), triglycerides, and blood pressure while raising your HDL (the good cholesterol) levels. Many studies show that soy is effective in relieving hot flushes, too.

Vitex (Vitex agnus castus)

Vitex, or *chaste tree,* acts like progesterone by helping to reduce perimenopausal stress and depression. (Some women find that it does just the opposite, but reports of vitex causing stress and depression are rare.) Because it acts like progesterone, vitex may help to stabilise the uterine lining. Herbalists say vitex is safe for long-term use.

Avoiding Problems with Plants

As we mention a lot in this chapter, just because herbs are natural doesn't mean that they're safe. People get into trouble with herbs because they don't realise that herbs are drugs that produce both positive and negative effects. Some people with certain medical conditions are more susceptible to the side effects associated with some herbs. For example, women with cardiovascular disease should take care with herbs because the containers don't necessarily carry any warning. Here are some other things to look out for when using herbs:

- ✔ Some herbs can damage your liver causing chronic hepatitis or acute liver injury. These herbs include chaparral, comfrey, coltsfoot, germander, Gordolobo yerba tea, mate tea, pennyroyal oil (also known as squaw mint), and many others.

- ✔ Therapies that contain the active ingredient *mefenamic acid* can cause liver and kidney damage (and sometimes your kidneys quit functioning altogether, which spells trouble).

If you feel heart palpitations or anxiety with any herbal therapy, stop using it immediately.

Getting Touchy about Acupuncture

Acupuncture is a form of traditional Chinese medicine. An acupuncturist inserts needles into specific points along critical energy paths in your body. For the doubters out there, acupuncture isn't all that far out. Asian doctors successfully perform surgery using acupuncture as the anaesthesia.

Acupuncture stimulates your body's ability to resist or overcome menopausal symptoms because it corrects energy imbalances. Acupuncture also prompts your body to produce chemicals that decrease or eliminate pain and discomfort.

Acupuncturists place fine needles into your body, which affect your *chi* – the life-force energy that travels through *meridians* – pathways in your body. Acupuncturists have mapped out the meridians and specific points along the meridians in the human body, so they know where to place the needle given your specific symptoms. You tell the acupuncturist your symptoms – heavy bleeding, headaches, and hot flushes, for example – and he or she knows exactly how to place the needles to relieve your discomfort.

Acupuncture is recognised as a legitimate form of complementary medicine. If you're interested in trying acupuncture, find a qualified specialist (see the Resources section in Appendix B).

Soothing Symptoms with Relaxation Therapies

Stress is great if it motivates you to do your best – in a race, for example. But, if you're continually stressed out, stress can cause physical damage to your mind and body. It can lead to excessive eating, sleeplessness, anxiety, depression, and irritability. (Do any of these symptoms sound familiar – as in perimenopausal and menopausal symptoms?) Continued stress can also affect your immune system, making you more susceptible to cancer, hypertension, heart problems, and headaches – some of the medical concerns that women worry about after menopause.

Take a look at some of the non-medical therapies that can help you relax and reduce the stress in your life.

Tuning in to biofeedback

Biofeedback is a technique in which body functions such as blood pressure, heart rate, skin temperature, brainwaves, muscle tension, or sweating are monitored while you try to change them using the power of thought alone. As you watch the monitoring device, and use trial and error, you discover how to adjust your thinking and mental attitudes to control bodily processes that people usually think of as involuntary. Using biofeedback, some people manage to control blood pressure, temperature, gastrointestinal functioning, and brainwave activity. Although originally championed by practitioners of complementary medicine, it is now widely used by medical doctors, too.

Some of the menopause-related conditions you can treat with biofeedback are

- Hypertension
- Migraine headaches
- Sleep difficulties
- Stress
- Urinary incontinence

Getting in your yoga groove

Now here's a great way to kill two birds with one stone: Yoga can help improve your flexibility (something that starts decreasing after living on this planet for about 35 years) and relieve stress. Yoga breathing exercises and postures have a calming action and help you to stay supple. Flexibility is an important part of balance, so flexibility reduces your chance of falling and breaking a bone. Reducing stress improves your immunity as it helps you to avoid disease and also to improve your mental outlook.

Yoga is also a great way to keep your bones strong and to improve your muscle tone. Yoga combines breathing, meditation, and stretching techniques to help strengthen bones and muscles and improve posture, breathing, oxygen flow, relaxation, and overall health and vitality. Take a yoga class or grab a book – try *Yoga For Dummies* by Georg Fauerstein and Larry Payne (Wiley). Many different forms of yoga are out there, and you should find this an excellent form of exercise for women of all ages.

Slip Sliding Away with Topical Treatments

Many perimenopausal and menopausal women experience *vaginal atrophy* (drying and thinning of the vagina). You can treat this condition in several ways without using hormone therapy.

You can buy lubricants without a prescription in pharmacies and supermarkets that help to relieve the day-to-day discomfort of vaginal dryness. A number of different ones are available, some of which are as effective as vaginal oestrogen cream in relieving vaginal dryness. Some come in a tube with an applicator. You simply fill the applicator, insert the tube into your vagina, and press the applicator. You repeat this process once a week.

In addition to over-the-counter lubricants, some of the herbs we discuss in this chapter also relieve vaginal dryness. (Check out the 'Cataloguing herbal therapies by symptom' section earlier in this chapter.)

If vaginal atrophy is causing painful intercourse, a number of lubricants are designed to help you get slippery. In fact, you may find that sex is more fun when you use a lubricant than it was before. You can rub any of these products on your vagina before intercourse. But, if using a latex rubber barrier method of contraception (condoms, diaphragms) check that the brand of lubricant you select is water soluble. Lubricants that are mineral-oil based quickly weaken latex rubber and are therefore unsuitable.

Chapter 17

Treating Common Menopause-Related Conditions without Hormone Therapy

. . . .

In This Chapter

▶ Beefing up your bones without oestrogen

▶ Heading towards a healthy heart without hormones

. . . .

*P*rolonged periods of low oestrogen levels promote bone deterioration and cardiovascular conditions. Although many women choose to use hormone replacement therapy (HRT) to prevent these issues, other medications and therapies that directly treat these issues are available. In this chapter, we look at treatments that target specific conditions and diseases. In contrast, hormone replacement therapy tries to treat these conditions indirectly as a result of adjusting hormone levels. Whether or not you use hormones, you can use the treatments you read about in this chapter. Some of the treatments are medications; others are lifestyle choices.

Battling Bone Loss and Osteoporosis with Medication

One of the best ways to avoid *osteoporosis* (brittle bone disease) is to start out with strong, healthy bones. You can accomplish this feat if you get plenty of calcium and vitamins D and K in your diet during childhood, adolescence, and early adulthood. (For the complete low-down on caring for your bones, check out Chapter 4.) Of course, hindsight is a wonderful thing, and it is possibly too late at this point in your life to start developing healthy bone mass. (But it isn't too late for the young women you know, so spread the word.) Fear not: In the following sections, we outline some other ways to improve the health of your bones during menopause without using HRT.

A number of drugs can help preserve bone density. The drugs we mention in this chapter, taken in combination with a healthy diet and exercise programmes, can slow your rate of bone loss and, in many cases, actually increase your bone density over time.

Beginning bisphosphonates

A group of drugs called *bisphosphonates* are effective medications for halting and reversing bone loss in menopausal women. These drugs slow down the destruction part (*resorption*) of the bone-maintenance process. Here are some examples of bisphosphonates:

- **Alendronate:** Also known as alendronic acid, this is one of the most commonly used bisphosphonates. It prevents bone material from breaking down, and actually builds stronger bones. When you include alendronate as part of a healthy lifestyle (enough calcium and regular exercise), you can cut your risk of fracture in half. Like all medications, alendronate comes with some rules. You have to:

  - **Take it first thing in the morning on a completely empty stomach.** You may have to adjust your morning schedule if you like to hop out of bed and into the coffee pot.

  - **Take it with a full glass of water.** Don't substitute coffee, juice, cola, or anything else. Use plain water.

  - **Remain upright after taking it.** Sorry, but you can't go back to bed. If you don't remain upright after you take alendronate, it can cause a burning sensation in your oesophagus.

  - **Wait for an hour after taking it before you eat breakfast.** Actually the longer you wait to eat or drink anything, the better your body absorbs alendronate. Waiting two hours before eating is even better than waiting just one. If you wait two hours, your body absorbs nearly 70 per cent of the drug, but if you wait only 30 minutes the percentage drops to about 46. If you eat when you take it, you don't absorb enough to help your bones.

  Alendronate comes in once-a-day and once-a-week pill form. Alendronate presents few side effects when you take it correctly, and those that occur are related mainly to indigestion, abdominal pain and distension. Women who are taking hormone therapy can use this drug to get even more protection against bone fractures.

✔ **Risedronate:** This bisphosphonate is supposed to have fewer gastrointestinal side effects than alendronate and has a slightly better track record in reducing the risk of fracture (65 per cent reduction in the risk of fracture for risedronate versus 47 per cent for alendronate). Risedronate comes in once-a-day or once-a-week pill form. You can take this medication even if you take hormone replacement therapy.

Considering calcitonin

Calcitonin nasal spray uses a different technique from the bisphosphonates to slow down bone loss. Calcitonin is actually a hormone that occurs naturally in your body. It helps to regulate your calcium levels as it slows down the rate of bone deterioration. It also relieves bone pain due to osteoporosis.

The rules with this stuff are simple but specific. You use one squirt in one nostril per day, alternating nostrils on a daily basis. (Is this a cruel joke or what? Don't the calcitonin bigwigs know that menopausal women often experience memory lapses?) Calcitonin isn't quite as effective at preventing bone loss as the bisphosphonates, but it may reduce the pain of existing spinal fractures.

Fathoming fluoride

All the bisphosphonates treat osteoporosis through a slowing down of the natural bone destruction process, but fluoride works on the other side of the bone-maintenance equation as it aids the formation of new bone. The bone built with fluoride is more brittle than normal, however, so although fluoride increases bone density it doesn't reduce fractures. After reading that statement, you may think, 'What good is thick bone if it's not strong?' Good question. That's why fluoride isn't normally used to treat osteoporosis. Some new research is using slow-release fluoride along with calcium supplements to see if stronger bone is built. Stay tuned for more.

Controlling Cardiovascular Disease

Cardiovascular disease includes conditions that affect your blood, blood vessels, and heart (otherwise known as the cardiovascular system). (For more on how this system works, see Chapter 5.) Controlling cardiovascular disease is the big one. Originally, HRT was thought to reduce the risks of cardio-vascular disease as one of the biggest benefits of HRT, but the results of the Women's Health Initiative (WHI) study have called all that into question. (See Chapter 11 for the low-down on this issue.)

The risks of cardiovascular disease are high for women after menopause – according to the British Heart Foundation, one out of every three women in the United Kingdom dies of some type of cardiovascular disease. And sadly, cardiovascular disease accounts for 24 per cent of premature death (before the age of 75 years) in women. Given the high incidence of cardiovascular disease in women over 50 and the controversy over whether HRT increases or decreases your risk, you *really* need to put some thought into how to keep your blood, blood vessels, and heart healthy for the next 40 or 50 years. In the following sections we provide you with some strategies.

Reducing your risk of heart attack

Half of all heart attacks occur in people with normal cholesterol levels, so a healthy cholesterol profile doesn't mean you're out of the woods. Of course, the other side of that story is that half of all heart attacks occur in people with lousy cholesterol profiles. So try to maintain a healthy diet and exercise programme and take your cholesterol medication if your doctor recommends it.

Atherosclerosis (clogged arteries) isn't the only problem that triggers a heart attack. Many other conditions can lead to a heart attack as well, including:

✔ Angina (blood vessel spasms)

✔ Arrhythmia (irregular heartbeat)

✔ Blood clots

✔ High blood pressure

To reduce your risk of heart attack, maintain a healthy diet, exercise regularly, and take the medication your doctor prescribes to treat high cholesterol and any other cardiovascular conditions. Your doctor may suggest one or more of the following to control or prevent heart attack:

✔ **ACE inhibitors:** Docs often use ACE inhibitors in people who have recently had a heart attack and who have heart failure or decreased function of the left ventricle. If used within 24 hours of the start of heart-attack symptoms, ACE inhibitors can stop you from dying from that particular heart attack and prevent heart failure stemming from the heart attack. The 'ACE' part stands for *angiotensin-converting enzyme*.

✔ **Aspirin:** Scientists have started paying a whole lot of renewed attention to this trusted pain reliever. The buzz surrounds aspirin's ability to lower the risk of heart attack, when taken every day. Aspirin performs this function as it keeps your *platelets* (special blood cells responsible for clotting) from sticking together too much and forming blood clots unnecessarily. Aspirin is an *anticoagulant* – it stops your blood *coagulating*, or clotting. If your body starts forming clots too readily, the clots can clog your blood vessels and lead to heart attack or stroke. If you have angina, your doctor may recommend aspirin to avoid a heart attack. If you've had a heart attack, your doctor may recommend that you take aspirin daily to avoid another attack.

Even though you can buy aspirin over the counter, it can have dangerous side effects. Read the warning label on the bottle and discuss possible side effects with your doctor. Preventing blood clots with aspirin can help you avoid a heart attack, but blood clotting is an important bodily function that stops you from bleeding if you cut yourself or have surgery. Therefore, always remind your doctor that you're taking aspirin regularly if you're facing surgery.

✔ **Thrombolytics:** Doctors give this class of drugs to patients having a heart attack due to a blood clot. Thrombolytics can rapidly dissolve a clot and restore blood flow to the heart. To work effectively, these drugs need to be given within six hours of the heart attack (before heart tissue begins to die from lack of oxygen).

✔ **Vasodilators:** These drugs help blood vessels to relax and dilate (widen) so that your heart doesn't have to work as hard to get oxygen-rich blood into the heart muscle. *Nitroglycerin* is a common vasodilator given to women who suffer from angina. Take these drugs as directed by your doctor.

✔ **Warfarin:** Doctors use warfarin to prevent blood from clotting but, unlike aspirin, warfarin is a prescription drug. Warfarin is more effective than aspirin in preventing blood clots, so you must use caution and have your blood monitored regularly when taking it. Women who have angina or who have irregular heartbeats often take this medication to help move blood more fluidly through the vessels.

Handling high blood pressure

A variety of drugs are available to treat hypertension (high blood pressure). They fall into a number of categories:

✔ **ACE inhibitors:** These block the enzyme angiotensin converting enzyme, or ACE, to encourage dilation of your small arteries and veins. This lowers blood pressure and increases loss of excess water and salts in the urine.

✔ **Angiotensin II blockers:** These are similar to ACE inhibitors but work one step further on, blocking formation of another substance, angiotensin II.

✔ **Beta-blockers:** These reduce your heart rate and blood pressure. Doctors also use beta-blockers to treat angina.

✔ **Calcium channel blockers:** These reduce your heart's oxygen requirements, increase the blood supply to your heart, and lower your blood pressure. They can prevent coronary artery spasms if you have angina.

✔ **Diuretics:** These are water tablets, such as thiazides, which flush excess fluid from the circulation.

Keeping your blood lean and mean

Blood that's high in LDL cholesterol (the bad stuff) and triglycerides encourages *atherosclerosis* – hardening and furring up of the arteries – and can eventually cause a heart attack (refer to Chapter 5 for the whole story). But some medications can lower bad cholesterol (LDL) and triglyceride levels and raise good cholesterol (HDL) levels, so:

✔ Get your blood cholesterol levels checked every year (total cholesterol, LDL, HDL, and triglycerides). Tests are readily available in chemists if your GP is reluctant to perform them on the National Health Service. For more information on blood cholesterol tests see Chapter 5.

✔ Visit your doctor regularly to assess your risk of cardiovascular problems.

✔ Read the labels on your foods and choose foods that are low in saturated fat and cholesterol.

✔ Keep your weight in check (turn to Chapter 18 for more on weighty issues).

✔ Exercise regularly (run over to Chapter 19 for some fab fitness recommendations).

✔ Don't smoke, and avoid second-hand smoke.

If changes in your diet, activity level, and lifestyle don't improve your cholesterol levels, your doctor may recommend medication to improve your cholesterol profile. Several types of drugs are available to lower cholesterol, but the main type used is the statins, which are very effective in lowering LDL levels by blocking an enzyme needed to make cholesterol in the body. Blocking this enzyme also lowers production of co-enzyme Q10 in the body, which may account for some of the muscle side-effects of the statins. If your doctor recommends that you take a statin, take co-enzyme Q10 supplements (60mg per day), too.

Your doctor is the only person who can determine whether cholesterol-lowering drugs are right for you and which type of drugs can meet your needs.

Living a hearty lifestyle

Here's a simple fact: Study after study has shown that smoking definitely increases your risk of cardiovascular problems because it promotes the build-up of fat and cholesterol in your arteries and increases the formation of blood clots that can cause heart attacks. Stopping smoking is a good way to lower your risk of cardiovascular disease. Your risk begins to drop immediately after you quit and, after your tenth anniversary of beginning a smoke-free life, your risk of cardiovascular disease is similar to that of a non-smoking woman.

Smoking isn't the only enemy of cardiovascular health. Weight matters. Gaining more than 8.16 kilograms (1 stone 4 pounds) after age 18 increases your risk of coronary heart disease, and your risk becomes greater as you gain more weight. If you've gained 18.1 kilograms (2 stone 12 pounds) or more since your 18th birthday, you've doubled your risk of heart disease.

A life full of anger, anxiety, depression, and isolation also increases your risk of cardiovascular disease. If one or more of these emotional conditions rule your life, it's not healthy, especially for your cardiovascular system. Having a network of friends or relatives who can offer you emotional support can lower your risk of cardiovascular disease. Try meditation or physical activity to reduce anger, depression, and anxiety. You should also share your symptoms with your doctor.

Picking a heart-healthy diet

Healthy eating guidelines recommend eating at least five servings of fruits and vegetables each day to reduce your risk of heart disease (and cancer). 'Get five to survive, but nine is divine' is a slogan used at the Cooper Institute, one of the most prestigious preventative-health institutions in the world. The institute is talking about the number of servings of fruits and vegetables you should consume *each day*. That means you need to spend less time in front of the dairy fridges and more time in the fresh fruit section at the supermarket. Five to nine servings of fruits and vegetables sounds like a lot, but meeting this goal is actually pretty easy. Check out Chapter 18 for dietary tips.

Part IV
Lifestyle Issues for Menopause and Beyond

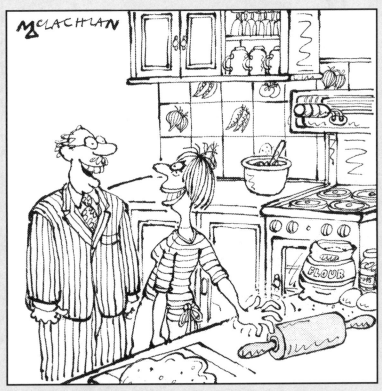

'You're looking <u>fantastic</u> these days – you must get the menopause more often.'

In this part . . .

Your body is changing. That's a fact. Your body is less forgiving about things like the pint of ice cream you just couldn't resist. That's a fact too. With all the changes going on, now is a perfect time to subscribe (or renew your subscription) to healthy habits like balancing your diet, getting a bit of physical activity, and breaking those bad-health habits. A few slight modifications in your daily routine can ensure that your body is living up to its potential. In this part, we offer practical advice that makes getting or staying fit before and after the change relatively easy. (And dare we say fun?)

Chapter 18

Eating for The Change

. . . .

In This Chapter

▶ Brushing up on good eating habits

▶ Using nutrition to alleviate health problems

▶ Reaching and maintaining a healthy weight

. . . .

*Y*ou've probably noticed that your body is less forgiving these days. In your twenties, you could order that extra glass of wine without paying for it on your hips the next day. Back then, over-exercising meant sore muscles the next morning; now it takes two days of ibuprofen, hot showers, and a massage to feel better. And an injury can set you back twice as long now as it did when you were a twenty-something.

Menopause is a natural reminder that your body is ageing and entering the prime time of nasty health issues. Lower oestrogen levels increase your risk of medical problems such as osteoporosis, cardiovascular disease, and more. A healthy diet and lifestyle can lower your risk for many of these medical issues, give you more energy, and improve your quality of life. It can also reduce some of the annoying symptoms of menopause, such as hot flushes.

Menopause gets your attention, up front and personal, with less than subtle physical reminders such as hot flushes, weight shifting to your middle, and heart palpitations. You can't help but take notice that your body is changing. If you're ever going to get in shape, now's the time. Indeed, now is the time to start your preventive healthcare programme so that you can continue to live a long, active, and healthy life.

You also need to address your eating habits as taking off weight is harder now than in the past. With middle age, your metabolism starts to slow down. If you also decrease your physical activity, which many women do when they reach middle age, you may find yourself gradually gaining weight. Lower oestrogen levels also trigger redistribution of fat so that it ends up around your waist. That curvy pear shape turns into more of an apple shape as fat migrates to your middle.

In this chapter we don't recommend any quick fixes. To stay healthy, you have to develop healthy *habits*. Habits are built on small changes that you can live with – without feeling as though you're making a tremendous sacrifice. If you adopt healthier eating habits, you can avoid dieting and feel better. Unfortunately we don't have a miracle programme, but we do suggest great ways to eat better so that you can get to a healthy weight, maintain that weight, and help reduce your risk of many diseases that strike menopausal women.

Eating to Promote Good Health

'You are what you eat' sounds trite, but scientific evidence shows that the foods you ingest affect your health. As junk goes in, health falls out, and you probably have real-life experiences that prove this point. During the major transformation that is menopause, you want maximum energy and protection from disease. A proper diet can help to ensure success on both fronts.

How do you promote good health through your diet? By adopting or maintaining healthy eating habits. Many studies link healthy eating habits to good health. *Healthy eating habits* means eating a balanced diet of foods that keeps your body well nourished and able to fend off disease and environmental toxins.

Studies show that people who eat at least five helpings of fruit and vegetables each day cut their risk of stroke by nearly a third and reduce their risk of cancer and heart disease. Research also confirms that the single most important factor in keeping the immune system healthy is a balanced diet.

Eating right helps your body fight off illness and protects your blood vessels, your bones, your heart, and other organs from chronic disease. Dieticians recommend that you eat at least five, and preferably eight to ten, servings of fruits and vegetables each day. The antioxidants, phytochemicals, and fibre present in fruits and vegetables build immunity, lower your blood pressure, and reduce your risk of heart disease, stroke, and many types of cancer.

Eating healthily is easier than you think. You don't have to walk around with a calorie-counting book. You don't have to eliminate all your favourite foods. You don't have to eliminate snacks. And you don't have to live on grapefruit juice and tofu. All you have to do is eat the right proportion of carbohydrates, protein, and fats and consume no more than 1,500–1,800 calories each day.

Sneaking in the vegetables

If you're not crazy about vegetables, try these easy and painless tips for fitting more vegetables into your diet:

✔ **Add vegetables to sandwiches.** Try lettuce, cucumbers, tomatoes, peppers, or bean sprouts. Remember you need only a handful of veggies to count as a serving.

✔ **Add chopped carrots, peppers, courgette, or yellow squash to shepherd's pie.** These veggies make tasty additions, and veggie-phobics barely notice them.

✔ **Add vegetables to your pasta.** Sauté garlic, onions, and chopped carrots or courgette in a pan sprayed with vegetable oil. When the pasta is tender, stir in the vegetables.

✔ **Combine a variety of colourful vegetables.** Try stir-frying (spray vegetable oil on the pan instead of pouring it from the bottle to lower the amount of oil you use), roasting (spray with vegetable oil and broil in the oven for 10 minutes), or barbecue (forget the vegetable oil altogether) the vegetables and then arrange them in colourful layers for visual appeal.

✔ **Add chopped vegetables to rice.** Peas, corn, broccoli, tomatoes, and peppers work well, but you can use any of your favourite vegetables.

Here's a quick example of a simple fruit-and-veggie meal plan that provides five of these great foods in one day:

✔ **Breakfast:** A piece of fruit with your meal

✔ **Lunch:** A salad or piece of fruit with your meal

✔ **Snack:** Another piece of fruit some time during the day

✔ **Dinner:** A vegetable and a salad, or two vegetables, with your meal

See how easy that is? Most people find quite a few fruits and vegetables that they like to eat, so turning your diet in a healthier direction is both fun and enjoyable.

Trendy diets come and go – and then come back again with a new name. Forget them. You don't need to follow the advice of a late-night, slick-talking, infomercial guru to eat healthily and achieve or maintain a healthy weight. A well-balanced diet keeps you full, and proper portion sizes along with exercise and planning keeps you at your preferred weight.

We list several great resources for eating healthily and losing weight, and keeping it off, in Appendix B.

Getting the right mix of nutrients

People eat for lots of reasons other than to satisfy hunger. You may eat when you're not hungry sometimes – perhaps for emotional reasons (you're bored, tired, angry, sad, or happy) or because certain environments trigger eating (you nibble as you clear the table, talk on the phone, or watch TV).

If you want to stay healthy and stick to a healthy weight, eat with a purpose! Think of food like fuel. The 'fuel' is your blood sugar, which gives you the energy to build muscle, repair cells, and fight illness. What do you need to keep your body fuelled during the day? You need to feed your body the right mixture of proteins, complex carbohydrates, and fats to keep your well-tuned machine purring. Table 18-1 shows the breakdown for a healthy, balanced diet.

Table 18-1	Balancing the Scales of a Healthy Diet
Nutrient	*Percentage of Daily Calories*
Protein	10–20
Complex carbohydrates	50–70
Fats	20–30

Proteins, carbohydrates, and fats work as a team to keep your energy level high and your body in good repair. Simple carbohydrates, such as sugar, give you quick energy, but this energy lasts only a few minutes. Complex carbohydrates, such as whole grains, fruits, and vegetables, fuel your body for up to three hours. Proteins provide energy over the course of four or five hours, and fats fuel your body for most of the day (five to six hours). Getting the right combination of foods throughout the day gives you energy and stops you having sudden cravings or feeling tired, anxious, or sleepy.

Scientists are researching *phytochemicals*, plant nutrients that may protect against heart disease and cancer and build your immune system. You find phytochemicals in all fruits and vegetables, especially red grapefruits, tomatoes, watermelons, lemons, and limes.

At any given meal, try not to include too much sugar (the energy you get from sugar lasts only 15–20 minutes, and you quickly become tired and hungry) or too much fat (fat provides lots of calories but not enough short-term energy). If you get the right combination of protein, carbohydrates, and fats, you'll be fully charged for three to five hours.

The best way to approach this nutritional trio is to eat foods belonging to each category during each meal. If you can't manage that, make sure that you achieve the proper proportion over the whole day.

In addition to eating right, try to drink plenty of fluids. Most dieticians recommend that you drink at least eight glasses of fluids a day, with at least four of those glasses containing simple water. If you're increasing the fibre in your diet, you may want to drink a couple more glasses of water each day to help the flushing process. Herbal teas and non-caffeinated, sugar-free soft drinks help you keep your fluids up without tacking on too many extra calories.

If you blow it one day, don't stress out. If you find yourself regularly struggling to eat the right amounts of the right foods, try sitting down and planning out your meals for a few days at a time. Paying attention to what you eat helps you control your eating and weight.

Fine-tuning your carb intake

The bulk of your diet should consist of complex carbohydrates, which works out well because fruits and vegetables – the food group you're supposed to eat five servings of each day – generally contain complex carbohydrates.

Simple carbohydrates

The quickest way to raise your blood sugar is to eat sugar (soft drinks, sweets, jam, and so on). It takes very little effort for your body to take sugar and put it into your bloodstream. As they quickly raise your blood glucose level, these simple carbohydrates are known as high-glycaemic foods.

Simple sugars give you a quick burst of energy, but your blood sugar drops just as quickly after about 15 minutes. Even athletes find that the quick rush of sugar doesn't do much to enhance their performance, so try to avoid these.

Complex carbohydrates

Think of complex carbohydrates as 'plant foods' because they include fruits and vegetables as well as wholegrains. You digest complex carbohydrates more slowly than simple carbohydrates, so they provide fuel over a longer period of time – up to three hours. As complex carbohydrates do not have a major impact on your blood glucose levels, complex carbs are known as low- or moderate-glycaemic foods.

Choose fresh fruits and vegetables over the canned or processed variety. The fresh versions contain more nutrients and fibre and less sugar and salt. Pick wholegrain products (flours, breads, cereals, and so on) over refined or processed grains because a lot of the vitamins, minerals, and fibre are in the outer layer (the hull) of the grain, which is removed during processing.

Fibre is a type of complex carbohydrate and is sometimes called *roughage*. Fibre is simply plant material that doesn't break down in the human digestive system.

- ✔ **Soluble fibre** dissolves in water and is found in a variety of berries and other fruits as well as oats, legumes, and potatoes. Because they pass more slowly through your digestive system, they keep you feeling full for longer.

- ✔ **Insoluble fibres** are not digested, so they act like brooms sweeping through your digestive system and ushering out those partially digested remnants from yesterday's meal. This type of fibre prevents constipation and improves a number of digestive problems such as diverticular disease and haemorrhoids (piles).

Try to eat eight or nine servings of high-fibre foods every day. Eating this number isn't as tough as it seems if you eat your vegetables and fruits and choose wholegrain breads and cereals.

Building with proteins

Proteins help build and repair cells, muscles, and tissues. Meat, fish, dairy products, peas, and beans are all high in protein. Most of these foods, with the exception of peas and beans, also contain high levels of fat and promote high cholesterol levels. (Refer to Chapter 5, where we explain about the dangers of too much cholesterol.)

To keep your body healthy while getting adequate amounts of protein, choose lean cuts of meat rather than the fatty stuff. Put fish or chicken on your plate more often than red meat. Nuts, seeds, pulses, cereals, textured vegetable protein (TVP) made from soya beans and mycoprotein, derived from a fungus, are also good sources of protein. Place low-fat milk products in your trolley instead of their whole-milk cousins. And limit your daily calories from protein to 10–20 per cent of your total intake.

Most people eat a lot more protein than they really need. You need only 120 grams (4 ounces) of protein a day. (A 120-gram serving of meat is about the size of a deck of cards.) A serving of fish or meat and a couple of servings of low-fat dairy products gives you enough protein for the day.

Energising with fats

Fats supply fatty acids that your body can't produce and help your body to absorb the fat-soluble vitamins A, D, E, and K.

Per gram, fats give you twice the energy of carbohydrates and proteins, but this means that they also contain *twice* the calories. High-fat foods are packed with calories and help you gain weight more quickly and easily than other foods. Fats also raise your cholesterol levels and increase your risk of cardiovascular disease, cancer, and diabetes.

You need a certain amount of fat in your diet, but you don't have to work to include it. Most people get far more fat than they need, which helps explain why more than half the people in the United Kingdom are overweight or obese.

Foods high in fats include both plant and animal foods. Here are just a few: fried foods, salad dressings, fatty meats (bacon, roast beef, lamb, pork, hot dogs, and more), dairy products (cream cheese, butter, ice cream, cheese, milk, and so on), pastries, nuts, and many other foods we love. (For more information on the dangers of fats and cholesterol when it comes to your cardiovascular system, please check out Chapter 5.)

Here's the low-down on the three basic types of fat:

- **Monounsaturated fats:** Although these fats are a bit more helpful than the others, you still need to keep monounsaturated fats under control as they contain lots of calories. These fats lower your bad LDLs and keep your good HDLs high. You find monounsaturated fats in peanuts and peanut oil, olives and olive oil, and avocados. A diet rich in olive oil reduces the risk of coronary heart disease by 25 per cent. An intake of around 2 tablespoons of olive oil per day is ideal (more if you're not watching your weight).

- **Polyunsaturated fats:** These fats usually come from plants. Corn oil, safflower oil, and many soft margarines fall into this category. Polyunsaturated fats lower your bad cholesterol (LDL), but they also lower your good cholesterol (HDL). Limit yourself to one tablespoon of polyunsaturated fats a day.

- **Saturated fats:** Found in butter, whole milk, meat, peanut butter, and pastries (among others), saturated fats elevate your cholesterol and triglyceride levels.

  Avoid eating saturated fats as much as you can. *Trans-saturated fats* ('trans fats') also raise cholesterol levels. You find these rascals in fried foods, bakery goods, ready meals, fast foods and other convenience foods, and certain margarines – look for spreads that have 'No trans fats' printed on their labels. Your heart will thank you.

Meals on wheels

You probably don't want to carry around a food chart that lists the nutrients and calories in every possible food you encounter throughout the day. The easiest way to plan and keep track of what you eat (without a chart) is to balance the portions of foods that you put on your plate. A simple way to do that is to think of your plate as a wheel sectioned into quarters.

Put vegetables and fruit on half the wheel, place a form of protein (fish, meat, chicken, beans,

and so on) on one quarter of it, and reserve the other quarter for a starch (such as a whole-wheat roll or brown rice).

Worried that there's no fat on your wheel? If you put a bit of dressing on your salad (on the vegetable half of your plate) or butter on your bread, your meal already contains plenty of fat. Remember that a little bit of fat carries a lot of weight.

Opt for polyunsaturated and monounsaturated fats over saturated fats and trans fats. And take advantage of the low-fat options that line the aisles of grocery shops. If you keep your consumption of fats down, you cut your risk of cancer.

Focusing on your feeding flow

To maintain a high level of energy and keep yourself charging ahead throughout the day, you have to put the right type of fuel into your tanks and maintain a continuous flow of fuel to your body.

To maintain your energy level, build muscle, burn calories, and balance your eating over the course of the day. Eat at regular intervals – approximately every three to six hours. If you follow this timetable, snacks actually play a key role in your daylong meal plan. They add the right types of food for balance and keep you from feeling deprived of food. Make sure that each snack contains fewer than 150 calories.

Some people eat only once a day. Why? They may take up this bad habit in an attempt to lose weight. Others claim that they don't have time to eat throughout the day. Whatever the reason, eating just once a day is a bad idea. If you only eat once a day, you're more likely to pig out when you do eat and get so stuffed that you feel tired and groggy after the meal. Eating just once a day doesn't give your body the nutrients it needs to burn calories and build muscle and tissue throughout the day.

Eating to Prevent or Contain Problems

Feeding your body the right foods can help to forestall certain health problems, and diet is part of the treatment regime for certain conditions. In this section we talk about the most helpful nutrients for health maintenance and prevention.

✔ **Antioxidants:** Ongoing research shows the importance of antioxidants in slowing the ageing process. *Antioxidants* eliminate free radicals from your body. *Free radicals* are to your body what rust is to your car: They promote damage to your infrastructure, leading to heart disease, lower immunity, cataracts, diabetes, and cancer. Antioxidants hook up with the free radicals and escort them safely out of your body so that they can do no harm. Colourful fruits and vegetables, such as broccoli, berries, grapes, pumpkin, and carrots, are especially high in antioxidants.

✔ **Fibre:** Fibre pushes food through your digestive system helping to protect your body against colon cancer, *diverticular disease* (formation of little pouches inside your colon), constipation, diarrhoea, haemorrhoids and other digestive problems. Fibre also helps lower your cholesterol levels and stabilises your blood-sugar levels. Importantly, fibre helps you lose weight as it gives you a full feeling that reduces appetite and hunger.

Fibre is found in the skins of vegetables and fruits and the outer layers of grains, so eating the skin of your baked potato and choosing wholegrains increases the amount of fibre in your diet.

✔ **Soy:** Researchers are just beginning to discover the benefits of soy. Soy may protect against breast cancer, heart disease, and osteoporosis. Soy proteins and isoflavones are *phytooestrogens* (plant oestrogens), which lower cholesterol and support your immune system. You can find soy in tofu, tempeh, soy milk, and soy yoghurt.

A single serving of soy per day is beneficial, but some research indicates that too much soy may affect hormone balance.

Strengthening your bones

Osteoporosis (brittle bones) is particularly common in women after menopause because long periods of lower oestrogen levels promote bone loss. To slow the rate of bone loss, try to have plenty of calcium in your diet and an adequate supply of vitamin D, which helps your body absorb calcium.

Diet and exercise are two of the best and easiest ways to improve the health of your bones. In the following sections we provide great suggestions for bone-healthy eating.

Feeding your calcium needs

Try to ingest between 1,200 and 1,500 milligrams of calcium each day (check out the table in Chapter 4 for your exact dosage). Break that down into an eating plan means you need to eat 500ml of dairy products, a glass of juice with added calcium, and two calcium-rich foods each day.

Many foods are naturally high in calcium, including dairy products (try to get the low-fat type) and green leafy vegetables such as spinach and spring greens. Many juices and breakfast products, such as cereal and frozen waffles, are 'calcium-fortified', making it even easier to add calcium to your diet.

Many women don't get enough calcium through the foods they eat and find it easier to take calcium supplements. If you're one of these people, take supplements (usually a pill or chewable tablet) divided into two or three smaller doses spread over the day, rather than in one large dose. By dividing the dose, you ensure maximum absorption of the calcium.

Calcium in the form of calcium lactate, calcium gluconate, calcium malate, and calcium citrate is most easily absorbed from the intestines. Calcium citrate is less likely to cause constipation than calcium carbonate and is also better for older people, who tend to produce less stomach acid.

Taking calcium supplements together with essential fatty acids, such as evening primrose and fish oils, increases the amount of calcium that is absorbed and deposited in bones.

Take calcium supplements with a glass of orange juice or tomato juice – the vitamin C helps you absorb the calcium as they are acidic. Taking calcium supplements with milk is also great because the lactose and vitamin D in milk also helps you to absorb calcium.

Here are a few good tips to help you get more calcium into your diet:

- If you eat cereal for breakfast, try the brands that have 400 or 500 milligrams of calcium in each serving. Instant oatmeal is also a good source of calcium but contains only about 100 milligrams of calcium in each packet.

- Add low-fat grated cheese to baked potatoes, salads, toast, and your favourite vegetables.

- Combine fat-free ricotta cheese with fat-free cream cheese and a squeeze of honey for a great bagel spread. You get more calcium and a very satisfying treat.

✔ Add non-fat dry powdered milk to oatmeal, casseroles, pancakes, yoghurt, and smoothies to bone up on calcium.

✔ Citrus juices with added vitamin D and calcium are easy to work into your daily routine and can give you much of the calcium you need each day.

✔ Some antacids such as calcium carbonate chews not only relieve indigestion but also contain 500 milligrams of calcium. They're worth a chew!

Absorbing helper vitamins

You need 10 micrograms (equivalent to 400 international units, or IU) of vitamin D each day to help your body absorb calcium. Try not to exceed 25 micrograms (1,000 IU) of vitamin D a day, because vitamin D is a fat-soluble vitamin, and is toxic if you get too much. Oily fish, eggs, butter, milk, cereals and low-fat spreads provide vitamin D, so you probably won't have too much difficulty meeting your daily requirements through a good breakfast.

You can get all the vitamin D you need from 10 to 15 minutes exposure to sunshine each day during summer, but not during winter in the UK. Sunshine stimulates your skin to produce vitamin D. Take a walk and kill two birds with one stone: Get your vitamin D *and* exercise!

Vitamin K is also good for your bones. Good sources are green vegetables such as lettuce, broccoli, cabbage, and spinach.

Potassium and magnesium are also critical in your quest to maintain bone strength. You can get these nutrients from greens (try spring greens and curly kale), beans, wholegrains, vegetables, and fruits.

Pumping up your cardiovascular system

Keeping your cardiovascular system healthy is a matter of keeping your blood lean and your vessels clean. Lean blood (low in LDL cholesterol – 'bad cholesterol' – and triglycerides) prevents the fatty deposits that can lead to all sorts of cardiovascular problems involving your arteries.

Curbing the fats in your diet and replacing them with fruits, wholegrains, and vegetables can help maintain healthy blood, arteries, and heart. The antioxidants, fibre, and other beneficial nutrients found in these plant foods help prevent cholesterol from oxidising and damaging your arteries and heart.

Fruits and vegetables deliver more fibre and complex carbohydrates and less fat than any other food group, which is critical to maintaining lean and clean blood. Also, the calcium, antioxidants, and other vitamins found in fruits and vegetables keep your blood, blood vessels, and heart healthy. Fruits and vegetables are 90 per cent water (low in calories) and very filling.

Watch those high-cholesterol foods such as egg yolks, sausages, bacon, ice cream, butter, cheese, pastries, fried foods, and fatty cuts of meat, as these foods can raise the cholesterol levels in your blood.

Keep an eye on your sodium intake if you're concerned about high blood pressure. One in three people in the UK has high blood pressure, even if they don't know it. Avoiding processed foods, smoked meats and fish, salty snack foods, canned vegetables, olives, pickles, and fast food can greatly reduce the sodium in your diet. Choose fresh vegetables and meats and low-sodium alternatives.

Weighing in on the Weight Issue

Most of us know that being overweight is unhealthy. Unfortunately, having excess weight in your menopausal years carries even greater health risks then in your youth.

The good news is that menopause provides the perfect opportunity to assess yourself and your goals near the mid-point of your life and get you started down the road to a new, healthier you.

Realising the perils of too much weight

Weight has an incredibly important effect on health. Overweight women are more likely than those who are not overweight to suffer heart disease, stroke, diabetes, and certain types of cancer. Overweight women are also more likely to die at a younger age. Body fat (measured by your body mass index – BMI – which we explain in the 'Finding a healthy weight' sidebar) is an even better predictor of your potential for health problems than weight. Studies show that the higher your BMI, the greater your risk of hypertension (high blood pressure). Menopausal women are already more susceptible to hypertension and other cardiovascular diseases (refer to Chapter 5 for more on healthy heart issues), so maintaining a healthy weight helps to keep your risk of cardiovascular problems as low as possible. Figure 18-1 shows you where you fall in relation to the target weight for your height.

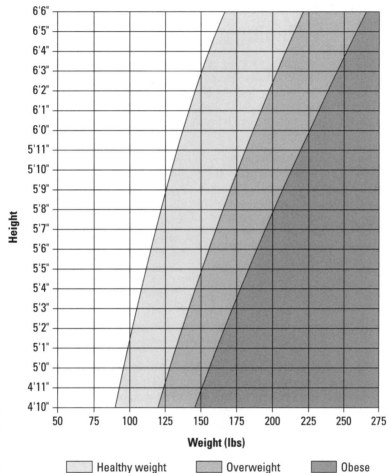

Extra weight not only collects around your middle after menopause but also raises your risk for a variety of unhealthy conditions such as high choles-terol, *atherosclerosis* (furring up of the arteries), heart disease, hypertension, diabetes, and stroke. Incidences of breast cancer, colon cancer, endometrial cancer, and gallstones also increase significantly in women who are over-weight during and after menopause.

One of the best ways to help your overall quality of life during and after the change is to maintain a healthy weight.

Finding a healthy weight

A *healthy weight* is a weight associated with people who have few health problems. You can find your recommended weight range from height and weight tables that are widely available. Your doctor or surgery nurse can let you know your ideal weight range, too.

You can fine-tune your health by evaluating your body fat. Body fat is the real villain in this story, not weight. To measure your body fat, visit your local health club and ask a member of staff to use callipers to measure the amount of fat in several places on your body. A general rule of thumb is that healthy women have between 18 and 27 per cent body fat.

Another measurement, your *body mass index* (BMI), which is based on your height and weight, provides a good estimation of body fat, and is easier to calculate. To determine your BMI:

1. Multiply your height (in inches) by itself.

2. Divide your weight (in pounds) by the number you arrived at in step 1.

3. Multiply your answer in step two by 705.

This is your BMI. If your score is under 25, you're in the healthy range. If your BMI is between 25 and 30, you are overweight, and women with a BMI over 30 (or if you're using a weight table – 20 per cent over your recommended weight) are considered obese.

A quicker way to see whether you're at a healthy weight is to look at Figure 18-1.

Your risk of *hypertension* (high blood pressure) increases when your BMI is above 20 and rises steadily as your BMI increases. Extra weight makes your blood vessels constrict. Even a modest weight gain of 2.3–4.5 kilograms (5–10 pounds) after menopause raises your risk of *hypertension* (high blood pressure). A study of thousands of nurses found that women who lost 4.5–9 kilograms (10–20 pounds) during the course of the study had a lower risk of hypertension than women who maintained a steady weight.

Because of oestrogen's role in maintaining healthy blood and vessels, your risk of cardiovascular problems rise after menopause as oestrogen levels fall. In addition, your risk of cardiovascular disease increases even more as your BMI increases.

Adult-onset diabetes leads to a slew of other medical conditions such as hypertension, circulation problems, skin ulcers, nerve disorders, stroke, blindness, heart disease, and kidney problems. If you've gained more than 5.4 kilograms (12 pounds) since you were 18, you've increased your risk of adult-onset diabetes; if you've gained more than 18.1 kilograms (2 stone 12 pounds), your risk of diabetes has gone way up. If you lose weight, you reduce your risk of diabetes dramatically.

Eating to control body weight

Many people struggle to control their weight, and no wonder! As a child you are encouraged to clean your plate if you want dessert, and advertisements promote over-indulgence of unhealthy foods that are 'naughty but nice'. The struggle to control your weight is a worthwhile battle, however. Achieving or maintaining a healthy weight has a tremendous impact on your overall health – and helps you look better and more youthful, too.

You don't have to quit eating your favourite foods. Just watch the size of your portions. Awareness is the first step.

Counting calories

To lose weight, you have to reduce the calories you eat and/or burn more calories through exercise. To maintain a healthy weight when you reach that point, you have to strike a balance between the calories you eat and the calories you burn through activity. But remember: You must get the proper nutrients to keep your body healthy and protect it from disease throughout the process.

Few people enjoy counting calories. If you're at a healthy weight and simply want to eat a healthier diet, just follow the advice in the 'Meals on wheels' sidebar. You will have more energy, suffer fewer food cravings, and help your body ward off disease and chronic medical conditions.

If your goal is to eat healthily to shed pounds, you need to focus on the calories you're eating and the source of those calories. Keep your calories within a healthy range, add a bit of exercise five days a week, and you can shed pounds while you improve your health.

Most people can eliminate lots of empty calories – the calories you eat without a purpose just because they're there. Do you ever finish up the chips on someone else's plate? Do you snack on leftovers as you clear the table? If so, you're falling into the empty-calorie trap.

Everyone is different, and your calorie needs reduce in later life. As a rough guide, here are the calorie recommendations for women:

- ✔ **To maintain your weight:** 1,500–1,900 calories a day
- ✔ **To lose weight:** 1,300–1,400 calories a day

If you're extremely active (exercising for more than an hour each day), add 100 calories to the recommendations.

Exercise burns up calories, so you can lose weight more easily and keep it off by incorporating exercise into your fitness plan. If exercise tips sound like a good thing at this point, check out Chapter 19.

If you're trying to watch your calories, take care with alcohol. Limit your alcohol intake to no more than three units of alcohol per week, where 1 unit of alcohol (10g) is equivalent to 300ml (half a pint) beer or 100ml wine (10 per cent alcohol by volume) or 50ml sherry or 25ml spirits. Wine and beer provide about 100 to 150 calories per unit.

The alcohol in a mixed drink is 100 calories or so, and if you mix it with something sweet you consume up to 400 calories per drink. Ouch!

Nibbling on little nothings

The following list provides good nutritional tips that have little or no caloric cost:

- Lettuce, parsley, radishes, watercress, and celery provide nutrients without the calories.
- Use butter-flavoured sprays instead of oil when cooking to shave off fat and calories.
- Sugar-free gelatin adds a bit of free dessert to any meal.
- Hot pepper and picante sauces add a bit of spice without a lot of calories.
- Low-fat bouillon is a great substitute for butter-based sauces when serving pasta or steamed vegetables.
- Fat-free cream cheese, mayonnaise, salad dressing, and sour cream are free in terms of fat calories as long as you use only 1 tablespoon at a time.

Foregoing fat

Many of our favourite foods are high in fat. Take away the fat, and some foods just don't seem so good. Believe it or not, meals can be *satisfying* without the fat. If you really dislike the low-fat alternatives, go ahead and have the high-fat food but reduce your portion sizes. Here are a few other great tips:

- Try mixing instant bouillon in hot water and adding a few tablespoons to vegetables, rice, or pasta instead of putting butter or margarine on the food. You get that rich taste without the fat.

Discouraging diets

It seems as if someone is always pushing a new diet that promises to make your weight disappear using a secret that no one else has discovered. Many of us try one of these 'miracle' diets and end up looking for a new one because the weight we lose reappears. The secret to getting to a healthy weight and staying there is to *avoid dieting* in the first place. Most diets have you chomping at the bit, waiting for the pounds to come off so that you can go back to eating the foods you want. When you go back to your old habits, the weight returns.

Eating healthier can help you lose weight and keep it off because it encourages you to change the way you think about food. You begin to think about food as a fuel, as opposed to a treat that you can't have or a substance that you must eat despite its cardboard-like flavour. You begin to think about what your body needs to stay lean, build muscle, rejuvenate tissue, and ward off disease.

Low-glycaemic diets, which avoid large swings in blood glucose levels, are good for weight loss and for reducing the risk of a number of health problems. Look for books that promote a low-glycaemic way of eating for health. Check out, for example, *The GL Diet For Dummies*, by Nigel Denby and Sue Baic (Wiley).

- ✔ Choose lean cuts of beef (tenderloin instead of rib-eye, for example) – they have less marbling than the fattier cuts.

- ✔ Try putting low-fat yoghurt or low-fat cottage cheese on top of your baked potato instead of butter or sour cream.

- ✔ When you order a salad at a restaurant, ask for the dressing on the side. If the restaurant doesn't have a low-fat alternative, try using just a tablespoon of a vinaigrette.

- ✔ Eat spicy toppings such as salsa, ginger, and picante sauce instead of cream sauces.

Chapter 19

Focusing on Fitness

. . . .

. . . .

*W*ith all the changes going on in your body, menopause is a great time to make sure that you're physically fit. Physical activity and exercise during perimenopause and menopause can relieve many of the common physical and mental/emotional symptoms that accompany the change.

We have good news: You don't need to have athletic tendencies or join a health club to realise tremendous health benefits from exercise. According to several studies, one hour of moderate exercise five times a week improves the quality and quantity of your life. In this chapter, we introduce you to exercises that you can do in your home and discuss ways to fit fitness into your busy life.

Maybe you're already physically active and you want to move your pro-gramme up a notch. If so, you're in the healthy minority: Studies indicate that only 20 per cent of women get 30 minutes of exercise five times a week. But we don't forget you if you have a head start on other women: In this chapter, we give lots of tips for everyone. You can see how your current fitness pro-gramme reduces your risk for many medical conditions and find suggestions to help you vary or supplement your routine.

Exercising to Enhance Your Menopausal Years

The lower oestrogen levels in your body during the change can contribute to a number of medical conditions, memory lapses, and emotional transforma-tions. Physical activity can help you reclaim your grip on life and fight off cardiovascular disease, diabetes, cancer, osteoporosis, and more.

The type of physical activity you need consists of movement that burns calories. Jogging or playing tennis burns lots of calories quickly, but seemingly mundane activities like vacuuming, gardening, and raking leaves are also beneficial if you do them for a long enough period of time (45 minutes to an hour). The trade-off is simple: Do a vigorous activity for a short period of time or a moderately demanding activity for a longer period of time.

Many studies show that physical activity makes a difference in the health of menopausal women. Exercise puts a positive spin on many of the health concerns you face during and after the change.

Adapting your attitude

A variety of studies show that exercise and physical activity improve your ability to cope with stress and depression. One study even shows that running is more effective than psychotherapy for reducing depression, and the results aren't that difficult to believe. The term *runner's high* isn't a joke – physical activity helps your body release *endorphins,* substances that naturally relieve pain and elevate your mood.

You can relieve your perimenopausal symptoms of anxiety, irritability, mood swings, decreased libido, and depression if you stick to a fitness plan that gives you time to build your mental and physical fitness.

Setting aside time for exercise each day also helps you to organise your thoughts and feelings, relieve stress and anxiety, and re-establish your grip on life. If you make the initial effort, you'll begin to look forward to *your* time.

Building up your bones

After menopause, you begin losing bone density. You risk developing *osteoporosis* (brittle bones) as a result of the loss. People who have osteoporosis are prone to fractures, which forces them to restrict their daily activity, which in turn impacts on the quality and longevity of their life. In Chapter 4 we give lots more info about osteoporosis.

To prevent osteoporosis and fractures, try following these suggestions:

✔ Include weight-bearing exercises in your physical routines to increase bone density (bone strength) and to slow or prevent bone loss. (See 'Strengthening bones and toning muscle' later in this chapter.)

✔ Improve your balance and flexibility with exercise that can help you to reduce your risk of falling and fracturing your bones. (Ease over to the 'Flexing through stretching' section later on for more information.)

Doing without diabetes

Diabetes is a serious health condition that produces a host of other medical problems ranging from hypertension to blindness. Exercise reduces your risk of adult-onset diabetes by keeping your weight in a safe range and improving your body's response to insulin and blood glucose levels. (For more on diabetes, see Chapter 14.)

Even if you're overweight or leading a sedentary lifestyle now, you can reduce your risk of diabetes if you begin a fitness programme. A small increase in activity helps, but more activity provides more protection from developing diabetes. According to one study, women walking briskly for three hours a week reduce their risk of diabetes as much as women who work out vigorously for half that amount of time, so you don't need to train for a marathon to reduce your risk of diabetes.

Flushing less and sleeping more

Only about 1 in 20 women who exercise experiences hot flushes. Compare that with the ratio of women in the non-exercising crowd who experience hot flushes – about one in four – and you see why tying up those trainers and going for a walk is a good thing. Hot flushes are a pain in their own right, but they can also turn into night sweats and cost you precious dream time. Exercise can lessen this effect and make your sleep more restful.

Exercise also helps you sleep better at night for another reason. Yes, exercise makes you tired, but there's more to the story than that. Exercise affects the amount of *melatonin* (a hormone that helps regulate sleep) in your body.

Melatonin levels are normally high in young children, but they appear to decline gradually with age in some adults. Exercise keeps the pineal gland producing melatonin at night (when levels are naturally higher), even though melatonin levels actually decline when you exercise.

Helping your heart

Just because a woman generally has the heart of a man ten years her junior because of the oestrogen her body produces, doesn't mean that heart disease doesn't catch up in the end. Keeping your heart healthy through diet, exercise, and medication, if necessary, is a priority for your menopausal years.

Cleaning up your cholesterol

Physically active women tend to have higher levels of the good cholesterol (HDL) than women who aren't so active. If you start exercising today, you can notice better HDL-cholesterol levels within a few months. Regular exercise also prevents the bad cholesterol (LDL) from building up and clogging your arteries. Check out Chapter 5 for the ins and outs of good and bad cholesterol.

Listening to your beating heart

Because physical activity improves your cholesterol profile, your blood vessels are less apt to play host to fatty build-up that results in atherosclerosis. Atherosclerosis leads to *hypertension* (high blood pressure), heart disease, and stroke, so getting physical reduces your risk of all three.

The Nurses' Health Study reveals that walking briskly for three hours a week can reduce your risk of heart disease by 40–50 per cent. This study also shows that even sedentary women who start doing a bit of regular walking benefit from a reduced risk of heart disease.

The more often you exercise, and the longer your work out, the more benefits you gain.

Keeping a lid on blood pressure

Because exercise improves your cholesterol profile, your risk of high blood pressure goes down too. With a healthier cholesterol profile, your blood vessels are less likely to get clogged with *plaque* (deposits of fat mixed with other substances that are covered with a layer of calcium and found on the walls of your blood vessels). Atherosclerosis causes your blood vessels to narrow and forces your heart to beat harder to get the blood through, raising the pressure in your blood vessels and resulting in hypertension (high blood pressure).

Exercising sound judgement

In case you haven't guessed by now, regular exercise seems to cure whatever ails you. This statement is especially true in relation to cardiovascular disease. Moderate exercise, such as walking for 30 minutes five times a week, can improve the health of your body and mind.

Exercise benefits your cardiovascular system in many ways. Working out:

- ✔ Improves your circulation
- ✔ Increases your good (HDL) cholesterol levels
- ✔ Reduces your total cholesterol, triglycerides, and blood pressure
- ✔ Increases your endurance
- ✔ Reduces your anxiety, depression, and emotional stress
- ✔ Builds a social group if you exercise with other people

Keeping clear of colon cancer

In Chapter 13, we discuss the benefits of having your colon checked regularly. Exercise is another way to protect yourself against colon cancer. Exercise keeps waste and any carcinogens you've ingested moving through your digestive tract and out of your body, so the nasties don't linger in your colon. An hour of exercise a day, five days a week, offers some protection against colon cancer too.

Living long and prospering

Even without gazing into a crystal ball, we say with confidence that daily exercise extends your life. One group of 60- to 80-year-olds cut their annual death rate in half just by walking two miles every day. Exercise can prolong both your quality and quantity of life by protecting against conditions as wide-ranging as hypertension, diabetes and haemorrhoids.

Sharpening your memory

Staying active as you age has a positive impact on memory and judgement. Getting more blood and oxygen flowing to your brain seems to trigger these positive effects. Keeping your brain active is also important, so read regularly, enjoy puzzles such as crosswords and sudoku or even spend time learning a new language.

Shedding pounds

Women typically gain about one pound a year from their late thirties through to their mid-sixties. A pound may not sound like much, but it adds up over the years. Weight gain raises your risk of many diseases. Women who incorporate 20–30 minutes of physical activity into their lives *every day* can maintain their present weight or lose weight. Even better is exercising an hour each day.

You can find all kinds of ways to lose weight, but to lose weight and keep it off, walking is one of the most effective physical activities. After studying thousands of dieters, one study found that 49 out of 50 people who lost 13.6 kilograms (2 stone 2 pounds) or more walked for at least half an hour at a brisk pace every day. The bonus: You don't need any equipment or special conditions other than comfortable shoes and personal motivation.

Focusing on the Fundamental Facets of Fitness

Whatever activities you choose to improve your physical fitness, make sure that you enjoy them. If you don't like an activity, you won't work it into your daily schedule and you won't do it for long.

Plan your week in advance to make sure that you reserve time for your workout. Make your fitness time a priority and don't give it up whenever things get busy. Working physical activity into your day helps you accomplish your primary long-term goal – living a long and healthy life – and makes you feel pretty good in the short term too.

Getting started

If you don't usually get much exercise, begin your programme slowly. For the first few weeks, exercise three times a week for about 20 or 30 minutes per session. Then, when you feel good with that pace and decide that you want to bump it up a notch, add a few more days and a little more time to your workout. Another way to move to the next level is to increase the intensity of your workout. If you're walking, go farther or faster or walk twice a day on certain days of the week. Or you may want to start jogging instead of walking. The bottom line: You gain more if you exercise longer or faster.

Regardless of how you decide to increase the intensity of your workout, make sure that your body gets used to each level before you move on to the next. If you start experiencing any abnormal symptoms, such as chest pain and unexplained shortness of breath, as you increase your exercise intensity, talk with your doctor.

Consider using your local health club, gym, or sports centre – these offer motivation, instruction, and an opportunity to form friendships with people who are also trying to stay healthy. But you don't have to join a club to receive these benefits: Asking a neighbour to join your morning walk or play a game of tennis also provides the support and motivation you need to stick with the exercise.

If you have any health problems, visit your doctor for a thorough physical examination before starting a new or more vigorous exercise programme.

Fitting in fitness

You may think, 'I don't have time to take a walk or work out'. We know that taking care of the approximately 12 million errands that your children, spouse, parents, and friends approach you with every day leaves you with little discretionary time or energy.

But fitness time is time that you devote to your health. Your family and your friends would agree that nothing is more important than your health. Besides, you're going to take time out of your life and away from your family and friends for your health whether you exercise or not. So, decide to take the time to exercise now or spend time with the medical professionals taking care of your health later.

Here are five simple ways to incorporate physical activity into an already busy day.

- ✔ Take the stairs instead of the lift. Whether you go up or down, you get your blood pumping and your legs working.

- ✔ When you're talking on the phone, stand up and stretch. Put your foot up on the table and stretch your hamstrings, do a few squats, bend from side to side, or walk around.

- ✔ When you go shopping, park your car away from the shops and walk briskly to your destination. When you're in a shopping centre, take a lap or two round the area. (Who knows? You may even spot a sale!)

✔ Make a permanent appointment with yourself to take a brisk walk first thing in the morning or after dinner each day – and make this walk the most important appointment of your day.

A walk first thing in the morning can help you to organise your day. An after-dinner walk can help you wind down from a busy day so that you sleep better. This is time that you devote to keeping yourself healthy so that your loved ones can hang onto you for longer.

✔ Use your lunch hour or break time at work to climb the stairs or take a walk around the building. On days when you can't get any other exercise, this break is sometimes the only time you have to get moving. Remember: Every little helps.

Planning your programme

After the onset of perimenopause, you want to keep your hormones balanced, your diet balanced, and yes, your fitness programme balanced. You should incorporate three types of activity into your fitness routine: aerobic exercise, flexibility training, and strength training. You're probably wondering how long this workout is going to take. Don't worry – you don't have to do all three each day, but you should fit all three in your weekly fitness plan.

✔ **Aerobic activity:** This form of exercise is great for your cardiovascular system. Aerobic activity increases your endurance and helps you to burn fat. Aerobic exercise is perfect for women of all ages. Whether you perform your aerobic activities in vigorous, relatively short bursts or at a slightly slower pace for longer periods of time, the benefits work out the same. For example, you burn 200 calories by walking for 30 minutes or jogging for 18 minutes.

Aerobic exercise benefits your body because it forces your cardiovascular system and muscles to exert themselves. Too little exertion and you don't gain all the benefits of exercise; too much exertion and you stress your cardiovascular system (and your muscles).

More vigorous forms of aerobic exercise include jogging, walking, cycling, aerobic dance, martial arts, and skipping with a rope. Even activities you probably don't think of as exercise can give you a light aerobic workout – walking your dog, golfing, shopping, gardening, and playing with the kids.

✔ **Flexibility training:** This aspect of your workout routine can protect you from injury, improve your balance, and provide muscle flexibility. Stretching is the simplest and easiest way to improve your flexibility and agility. Working with a *Swiss ball* (an inflatable ball about two to three feet in diameter) improves your flexibility and balance while strengthening and toning your muscles. Yoga is probably the oldest form of stretching.

✔ **Strength training:** Incorporating strength training into your exercise schedule helps you build muscle tone, endurance, and bone density. Because strength training builds muscle, it speeds up your metabolism so that you burn more calories – even when you're resting. (Muscle burns more calories than fat so the more muscle you have, the more calories you burn.)

Scheduling fitness fun time

A total fitness programme incorporates aerobic exercise, flexibility training, and strength training in a weekly fitness plan. In this section, we suggest a balanced programme incorporating all three training elements.

The plan includes two rest days each week (preferably not back to back) and one easy day. On the other days, try to give your best – work out at a comfortable but challenging pace. Breaking your workout into two or three sessions during the day because of time constraints is fine. And you can modify your days to suit your personal preferences.

Always warm up before each session and cool down afterwards. (For more information, see the 'Warming up and cooling down' section in this chapter.) In the fitness programmes we mention here, stretching forms part of the warm-up and cool-down routines, but you can add more stretching to your programme or add a yoga class to your schedule. Stretching improves flexibility and keeps your muscles from getting sore.

Start your fitness calendar on whatever day of the week makes sense to you. Many people start on Monday to coincide with the work week. Doing so with the routine outlined here lets you start your week with a good workout and end it with a rest day. Or maybe you're the type of person who prefers to start your week slowly and increase your level of activity as you go. You decide.

✔ **Day 1:** Assuming that you like to hit each new week running, start off Day 1 with a warm-up. Then move on to 20 to 30 minutes of aerobic activity followed by 20 minutes of strength training (see the 'Strengthening bones and toning muscle' section later in this chapter). End your workout with a cool-down that includes at least 5 to 10 minutes of stretching.

✔ **Day 2:** Do 20 to 30 minutes of aerobic exercise but at a lower intensity than your Day 1 workout. Remember your warm-up and cool-down time.

✔ **Day 3:** Do the Day 1 routine – warm-up, aerobic exercise, strength training, and then a cool-down with good stretching. Your intensity is the same as that of Day 1.

✔ **Day 4:** Take a day off to rest and restore your muscles. Resting is also important for your body.

✔ **Day 5:** Follow the same workout as Days 1 and 3.

✔ **Day 6:** This is ladies' choice day. Do something different for your aerobic exercise, something a bit lighter – gardening, dancing, swimming with the kids, or golfing – but do it for 45 minutes rather than a half-hour.

✔ **Day 7:** Take the day to rest and relax to restore your muscles.

Creating a Personal Fitness Plan

Planning is essential. If you don't have a plan, making something happen and tracking your progress is hard. Start slowly and work your way up to more intense, more frequent, and longer lasting workouts. You can also incorporate some of the strength training and flexibility training exercises into your weekly workout.

If you haven't exercised in a long time, if you have heart disease, if you're overweight, or you have any other medical condition, talk to your doctor about your fitness plan or find an experienced personal trainer to guide you.

Flexing through stretching

You probably stretched back in the days when you did gym at school, tried ballet, or ran track races, but things have changed a bit. In the past few years, medical and exercise experts have come a long way in understanding the physics behind stretching. Some of the old stretching exercises actually hurt your body more than they help. So read on for good advice about stretching. (And check out Figures 19-1 to 19-6 in the next section for a great introductory stretching routine.)

✔ Don't bounce. Stretch slowly until you feel tension, not pain.

✔ When warming up, hold the position for 10 to 30 seconds, relax, and then stretch again.

Zoning in on your target heart rate

The best way to make sure that you're doing enough exercise to benefit your health and your heart is to check your *heart rate* (how fast your heart is beating). Your heart rate tells you how much effort you put into an exercise. Here's how you can check your heart rate:

1. Put your index and middle finger on your opposite wrist and find your pulse. (You can also use the carotid artery in your neck, which is under your jawbone.)

2. Count the number of beats for ten seconds (you need a watch with a second hand).

3. Multiply that number (the number of beats in ten seconds) by six. The result is your number of heartbeats per minute – your heart rate.

After you know how to figure out your heart rate, you can figure out your *target heart-rate zone,* which is important when exercising. Try to keep your heart rate within your target heart-rate zone during exercise to achieve the perfect workout intensity and maximum benefits.

1. Subtract your age from 220, which is the maximum heart rate (a heart rate you don't want to even approach).

2. Multiply your answer from Step 1 by 0.6. The resulting number is the lower limit of your target heart-rate zone.

3. Multiply your answer from Step 1 by 0.85. The resulting number is the upper limit of your target heart-rate zone.

✔ When cooling down, hold the position for 30 seconds, relax, and then stretch again. If you're working on flexibility, try doing each stretch twice during the cool-down and stretch a bit further the second time.

If you increase your stretching intensity during the cool-down period when your muscles are already warm, you can increase your range of motion and get more out of your stretch. Stretching when your muscles are warm helps you to build flexibility much more quickly because warm muscles stretch better than cold ones, and elastic and stretched muscles are flexible muscles.

✔ Never stretch a muscle if you've had a recent muscle, ligament, tendon, joint, or bone injury or if you feel a sharp pain. If you feel a sharp pain – as opposed to the dull ache of well-exercised muscles – consult your doctor before continuing with your stretching routine.

If you're interested in additional information on stretching, take a look at the resources in Appendix B.

Yoga is a terrific activity if you really want to work on your flexibility and balance. Yoga consists of three main components: exercise, breathing, and meditation. Over a hundred different schools of yoga exist, so find the type that suits your objectives.

Like any physical workout, begin slowly and be patient with yourself. If you're interested in finding out more about yoga, check out the resources in Appendix B at the end of this book.

Warming up and cooling down

Be sure to start *each workout* with an easy warm-up period and end each session with a cool-down period. Warming up puts your muscles and cardiovascular system on alert that they're about to go to work. Cooling down gives them a chance to relax after a satisfying workout. You can do the same activities for both your warm-up and cool-down sessions.

Warming up and cooling down is sometimes as simple as walking or cycling for four or five minutes and then doing some *light, gentle* stretching for another five minutes.

Never stretch cold muscles – you can damage them. That's why you start your warm-up session with a bit of walking or cycling. Also, don't bounce or pull hard as you stretch during your warm-up, a time when your muscles are still pretty cold.

If you're short of time, you may be tempted to skip your warm-up and jump right into your routine. Not a good idea! Warming up prevents injury and helps you to ease into your workout without straining your muscles. Starting slowly actually lets you exercise longer.

The six simple stretches we show in Figures 19-1 to 19-6 stretch all your major muscle groups. Try holding each stretch for 10 to 30 seconds. Over time, you may want to try to stretch further, which is great, but don't strain your muscles and always stop when you feel tightness – don't stretch until you feel pain. If you stretch until you hurt, your muscles actually begin to contract, and you don't accomplish anything except hurting your muscles.

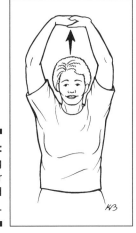

Figure 19-1:
Stretching
your upper
torso and
arms.

1. Clasp your hands above your head, interlocking your fingers.

2. Push your palms upward.

3. Stretch until you feel tightness and hold.

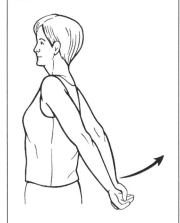

Figure 19-2:
Stretch-
ing your
chest and
shoulders.

1. Clasp you hands behind your back.

2. Slowly and carefully lift your arms.

3. Stretch until you feel tightness and hold.

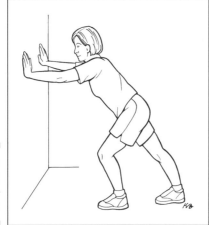

Figure 19-3:
Stretching
your legs —
all the way.

1. Stand close to a wall with one leg forward.

2. Bend your front leg at the knee and keep your back leg straight.

3. Steady yourself by putting your hands on the wall.

4. Stretch forward keeping your back foot (including your heel) flat on the floor.

5. Switch legs and repeat Steps 1 through 4.

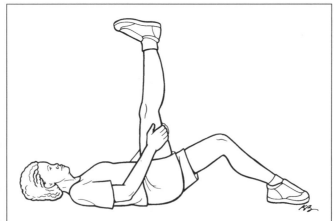

Figure 19-4:
Stretching
more of
your legs.

1. Lie flat on your back.

2. Stick one leg up in the air.

3. Grab your thigh below your knee.

4. Slightly bend the leg that is on the floor at the knee.

5. Gently pull your leg toward your chest keeping this leg straight.

6. Repeat Steps 1 though 5 with the opposite leg.

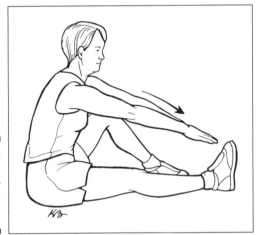

Figure 19-5:
Stretching
your lower
back and
buttocks.

1. Sit on the floor with both legs extended straight out in front of you.

2. Bend one leg so that your knee touches your chest.

3. Lean forward, reach out, and touch your toes.

   If you can't touch your toes, stretch as far as possible without experiencing pain. With time, you'll get closer and closer.

4. Repeat Steps 1 through 3 with the opposite leg.

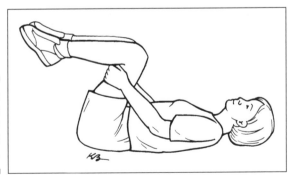

Figure 19-6:
Warming up
your lower
back and
upper legs.

1. Lie on your back.

2. Raise your legs in the air and bend them at the knee.

3. Grab both legs behind and below the knee.

4. While keeping your back as flat to the floor as possible, pull your thighs in toward your chest.

A lot of people tend to cheat at the end of their workout, but definitely do some light stretching as part of your cool-down – stretching is terrific for your flexibility. You can stretch further and more easily after your muscles are really warm from prolonged exercise. You can make great strides in your flexibility and agility if you do five or ten minutes of stretching after your workout.

Exercising to Overcome Osteoporosis

The best exercises to prevent or slow down osteoporosis are *weight-bearing exercises* – exercises, such as walking and strength training, that include gravity and tension on your muscles. Stress builds bone (aha – stress is good for something after all!), and putting weight on your bones provides the stress your bones need to grow in strength. Weight-bearing exercise promotes bone growth, which is critical for women of any age. During and after the change, when your oestrogen levels are lower, weight-bearing exercise can keep bones strong and healthy by increasing bone density.

Although you move your muscles when you swim or cycle, these aren't the best exercises for building bone. The water (in swimming) and the bicycle seat (in cycling) take a lot of the load off your bones.

If you have osteoporosis, your bones are more liable to break. Weight-bearing exercises are great for strengthening bone, but increasing your flexibility and balance can also help you to avoid osteoporosis-related complications by reducing your risk of falling and breaking bones in the first place. You can improve your flexibility if you include stretching in your fitness routine (check out the two preceding sections). And you can improve your balance through exercise as well.

The following sections discuss strength training and balance exercises – two types of exercise that can help you fight osteoporosis and osteoporosis-related complications when incorporated into your fitness programme. (For more information on walking, another weight-bearing exercise that, like strength training, can help you build bone, check out the 'Walking your way to fun and fitness' section later in this chapter.)

Strengthening bones and toning muscle

Walking is a great way to fight osteoporosis, but a combination of walking and strength training is even better for building bone. You may choose to do both of these weight-bearing exercise routines on the same day or split them up during the course of the week – whatever your schedule allows. Weight-bearing exercises strengthen only the bones that you work, so walking strengthens your legs but not your other bones. You need to introduce strength training exercises into your fitness programme to help your other bones.

The best strength training programme is one that includes all your major muscle groups. This type of programme improves your bone density in important areas, but it also improves your balance, which is important in avoiding falls that can cause fractures.

Start your strength training regimen with a good, all-round strength training routine using the seven exercises shown in Figures 19-7 to 19-13. These exercises strengthen your chest, arm, shoulder, leg, abdominal, and back muscles. You can start with three to five repetitions of each exercise and increase the number as your interest and endurance dictates. If you want to vary this routine or try more advanced strength training exercises, check out Appendix B for additional resources.

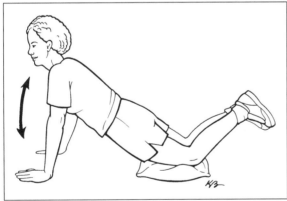

Figure 19-7: Push-ups for beginners.

1. Kneel on the floor (using a cushion if you have dodgy knees).

2. Place your hands a little wider than shoulder-width apart on the floor in front of you.

3. Keeping your knees on the floor (or on a cushion on the floor), raise your feet a bit.

4. Lower your upper body by bending your elbows.

5. Push back up and straighten your elbows.

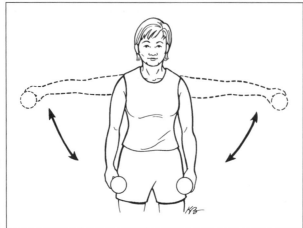

Figure 19-8:
Lateral
raises.

1. Stand up straight with your chest out and knees slightly bent.

2. Hold a 1-kilogram weight in each hand with your arms down at your side.

3. With your elbows slightly bent, raise your hands to shoulder level. (Don't raise them higher than shoulder level.)

4. Slowly lower your hands until the weights are back at your side.

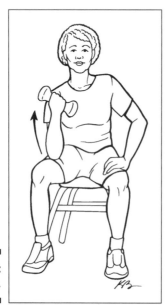

Figure 19-9:
Bicep curls.

1. Sit on the edge of a chair with your back straight and your legs slightly apart.

2. Lean forward (keeping your back straight).

3. Bend your elbow toward your chest and place it on the corresponding thigh while holding a 1-kilogram weight. (You can increase the weight as you get stronger.)

4. Slowly lower your arm by straightening out your elbow. (The palm of your hand should be facing up at the end of the motion.)

5. Bring the weight back toward your chest.

6. Repeat Steps 1 through 5 with your other arm.

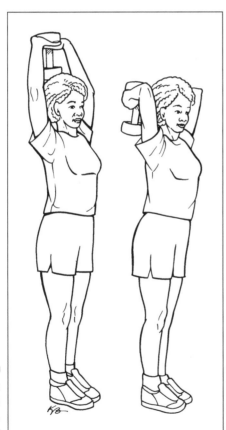

Figure 19-10:
Triceps
curls.

1. Stand up straight with your knees bent slightly.

2. Hold a 1-kilogram weight with both hands and raise it over your head.

3. Keeping your arms close to your head, lower the weight behind your head by bending your elbows.

4. When your forearm touches your upper arm, slowly raise the weight back up.

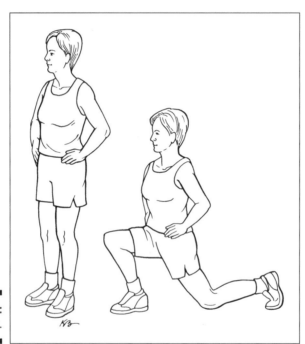

Figure 19-11:
Lunges.

1. Stand up straight with your hands on your hips.

2. Step forward with your right leg, keeping your back, neck, and head straight.

3. As your front heel hits the ground, bend both knees so that your left knee almost touches the floor (or go as low as you can).

4. Step back to the starting position.

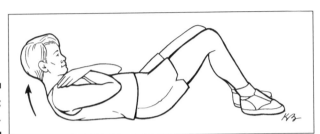

Figure 19-12:
Crunches.

1. Lie on your back with your arms crossed over your chest and both legs bent so that your shoes rest flat on the floor.

2. Slowly lift your upper body until your back is flat on the floor.

Don't just lift your head or you'll exercise your neck instead of your abdomen. And don't strain to pull your upper body farther up – just pull until your back is flat on the floor.

3. Relax and slowly lower yourself back to the floor.

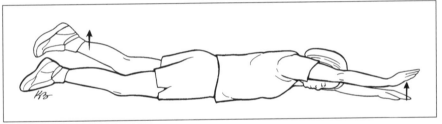

Figure 19-13:
Back
extensions.

1. Lie face down on the floor with both legs straight out behind you and both arms straight out over your head with your palms facing down.

2. Keeping your knees and elbows as straight as you can and your hips, tummy, and forehead flat on the floor, slowly lift your right arm and your left leg at the same time.

Don't laugh! Back extensions are not as easy as you may think.

3. Switch sides and lift your left arm and right leg at the same time.

Bringing balance into your routine

To avoid falling and possibly breaking a bone, spend some time working on your balance. You can challenge the muscles that keep you balanced in many fun ways, and you can tone your muscles at the same time. Talk to a personal trainer to find out more about the following exercise aids:

- ✔ **Balance board:** Stepping on this board feels like jumping on a moving surfboard after drinking three glasses of wine. Essentially, a ball is attached to the bottom of the board to challenge your balance (to say the least). As you strengthen your 'balance' muscles with this contraption, you improve your overall sense of balance and your muscle tone.

- ✔ **Exercise tubing:** If your friends and family see you with this tubing, they'll think that you're playing with a giant rubber band, so you may want to use this exercise aid in private. Exercise tubing is used in conjunction with stretching to increase flexibility.

- ✔ **Fitness balls:** Sometimes called Swiss balls and exercise balls, fitness balls are popular because they help you strengthen the *core balancing muscles* (abdominal, back, and hip muscles) that you use in many everyday activities.

  If you're up for a challenge, sit on a fitness ball and try to lift your feet. You can work up a sweat, exercise your abdominal muscles, and feel like a seal in a sideshow all at the same time. You can use these balls in a million different ways to improve both your balance and your muscle tone. *Exercise Balls For Dummies* by LaReine Chabut (Wiley) is a good place to start.

All these props can help you to improve your balance, flexibility, and strength. You can use them at home or in your health club.

Exercising to Protect Your Heart

A balanced fitness plan keeps you healthy after menopause. Aerobic exercises are perfect for reducing your risk of hypertension, heart disease, stroke, atherosclerosis, and other types of cardiovascular disease. These exercises, which are the core of a good cardiovascular workout, increase your blood circulation, strengthen your heart muscles, and improve your cholesterol profile.

Working on and working up to heart health

You can choose from any number of great aerobic sports or activities to improve your fitness. Cycling, jogging, swimming, dancing, and stair climbing are a few examples. If you want to vary your workout, try an aerobic activity other than walking or check out the resources in Appendix B that have more info on starting a fitness plan.

The following 'Walking your way to fun and fitness' section outlines a walking regime, which is an excellent way to begin your cardiovascular workout. Incorporating stretching and strength training into your aerobic workout provides variety to keep things fun (and ensures that you don't quit your aerobic routine because it becomes monotonous), increases your cardiovascular endurance, and allows you to quicken your pace. Try to work your way up to a routine similar to the one we lay out in the 'Scheduling fitness fun time' section earlier in this chapter.

As you improve your cardiovascular fitness, you feel less tired when you work out even though you're doing the same amount of exercise. You also notice that your heart rate gradually decreases, both during exercise and when at rest.

Build your endurance and stamina slowly. Don't overdo it when you first begin an exercise programme. Always stay within your *target heart range* (see the 'Zoning in on your target heart rate' sidebar in this chapter). If you're a beginner, keep to the lower end of your target range until you establish a comfortable workout plan. You can lower your risk of heart problems associated with exercise if you monitor your heart rate. To get the most out of your aerobic exercise, exercise at your target heart rate for at least 20 minutes.

A simple way to check whether your workout intensity is appropriate is the *walk-and-talk test*. If you're exerting yourself but you can still carry on a conversation while you exercise, you're probably exercising at the right pace.

Exercise is the best gift you can give your cardiovascular system. Just 30 minutes of walking five or more times a week can effectively improve your cardiovascular health. All you need for walking is a comfortable pair of shoes and 30 minutes. If you need to break your workout up into two 15-minute sessions or three 10-minute sessions during the day, don't worry; it still works, and provides the same health benefits.

If you want to continue to build your cardiovascular fitness, increase the intensity of your workout by increasing the

- ✔ Distance
- ✔ Speed at which you work
- ✔ Time you spend doing the activity
- ✔ Number of days you exercise each week
- ✔ Level of difficulty of your course (if you're a walker or cyclist, find a hillier course; if you use a treadmill, increase the incline or spend time on a stair-climbing machine)

As you increase the intensity of your workout, your cardiovascular fitness improves and you burn more calories. But, when you make your workout more challenging, do it slowly and take one step at a time. For example, you may choose to exercise at the same pace but add another half a mile to your walk. Try the new distance out to make sure that you're not going to get sore.

Walking your way to fun and fitness

As an exercise of choice, walking is perhaps the easiest way to begin a fitness programme. You don't need any equipment – just the will to get moving. Before you put your feet to the pavement, map out a route to follow on your daily trek. Here are a few pointers:

- ✔ Measure out a 2-mile course that you can easily expand to a 3-mile course when you want to increase the length of your walk.
- ✔ Pick a pretty area in your neighbourhood, around your workplace, or in a local park, or find a local running track (although circling a track can get *very* monotonous).
- ✔ Make sure your route is conveniently located. You don't want to give yourself the 'it takes too long to get there' excuse.

For the first two weeks of your new walking regime, walk the 2 miles three times a week and time yourself. Set a pace that's brisk enough to get your heart pumping, but not too fast that you can't talk and breathe at the same time. A good pace for many people is to walk 2 miles in about 35 minutes. During Weeks 3 and 4, step up your programme a bit. Walk four times a week instead of three. And try to increase your pace – do your 2 miles in half an hour.

At this point in your exercise progression, you need to check yourself and see how you feel. How easy was the transition from Weeks 1 and 2 to Weeks 3 and 4? Do you feel like you can do more or are you comfortable with your current routine? Depending on your age and your health, you may want to stick with this walking schedule for a while. When you feel your body getting stronger and your outlook is ready for another challenge, move along to the next level. (For the sake of simplicity, this section uses a weekly progression to outline this entire schedule. But remember that your Week 5 doesn't have to start until you feel ready for it.)

During the course of the next four weeks, your goal is to walk 3 miles five times a week. Work up to this goal slowly. Add ½ mile to your distance during Week 5. At that point you're walking 2.5 miles four times during the week. Then, for Week 6, walk 2.5 miles again but try to walk five times this week instead of four times. Keep your pace brisk.

If you're ready to go on after Week 6, charge ahead and add another half mile to your distance and walk five times this week. By Weeks 7 and 8, you're at your goal of walking 3 miles, five times a week. But just because you've reached this goal doesn't mean you can't aim higher. The important thing is that you find your comfort level. Many people are fine with this workout level for the rest of their lives – it can boost your spirits and your health.

Want to take your programme further? You've got the idea now – simply add distance, go faster, or make the course harder (try hills). If you have to miss a workout, get back on track as soon as possible – good habits are hard to break!

It may take you three or four months to reach the goal of 3 miles, five times a week – and that's fine. Walking is not a contest. You're doing it for yourself and your health. Your only opponent is inactivity.

Part V
The Part of Tens

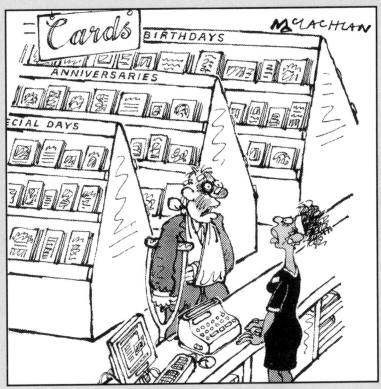

'Have you got a card for someone who's going through a very bad menopause?'

In this part . . .

This just wouldn't be a *For Dummies* book without a yellow and black cover and a Part of Tens. We like to think of the Part of Tens as the icing on the cake – better yet, the fat-free whipped topping on the bowl of fruit. If you like top-ten lists, you've come to the right part of the book. In this part, we expose myths about menopause, give you the scoop on medical tests that you may run into, and outline some great ideas and programmes that you can use to kick-start or jazz up your exercise routine.

Chapter 20

Exposing (More than) Ten Menopausal Myths

. . . .

In This Chapter

▶ Ferreting out the realities of menopause

▶ Keeping sex sexy after the change

▶ Determining the accuracy of blood tests

. . . .

A recent survey shows that half of all women going through the menopause feel unprepared and uninformed to face the change. Check out the following common menopause myths and see how many you know – and how many you simply bought into. Because menopause and misconceptions go hand and hand so often, we list a few more than ten myths in this Part of Tens chapter.

You're Too Young for the Menopause in Your Thirties and Forties

Not really. Even though most women reach the menopause sometime between 45 and 55 years of age (the average age is 51), going through menopause earlier isn't impossible or unheard of. Making the situation seem even less cut and dry are those annoying symptoms, such as hot flushes, crying spells, mood swings, and interrupted sleep, that usually occur years before you actually quit having periods (official menopause). Those physical changes that characterise what most people refer to as 'the change' are really more characteristic of *perimenopause* (the period of fluctuating hormone levels leading up to menopause). Some women experience perimenopausal symptoms for a decade before the onset of menopause. So having hot flushes and fertility issues in your late thirties and early forties is perfectly normal.

But keep your doctor informed about your periods because skipping periods during your late thirties or early forties can also indicate medical problems. For some women, certain medical treatments cause the early onset of menopause, for example:

- ✔ Chemotherapy or radiation treatment may cause your ovaries to shut down early, depending on the type of treatment.

- ✔ If you have both your ovaries removed, you immediately experience *surgical menopause.* The ovaries, responsible for producing the active form of oestrogen that serves many bodily functions, are gone, and menopause begins.

- ✔ *Autoimmune disorders* (diseases of your immune system) and thyroid problems can result in *premature menopause* (menopause before age 40).

If you go through menopause earlier than most women, you may also increase your risk of developing menopause-related medical conditions, such as osteoporosis and cardiovascular disease, earlier than normal. So talk to your doctor about ways you can prevent these conditions.

Menopause Is a Medical Condition that Needs Treatment

Not exactly. Remember puberty? Well menopause is puberty in reverse, with all the accompanying physical and emotional changes. (Sounds like a lot of fun when put that way, eh?) Menopause isn't a medical condition in that menopause is not a disorder. It's a natural passage from your reproductive years to the rest of your life.

Menopause isn't a condition that requires medical attention any more than puberty requires medical attention. (The same degree of patience, however, is required.) The changes that take place are normal and natural. The care you receive on your journey through menopause is meant to alleviate your discomfort and prevent disease rather than interfere with the natural process. Many women don't experience any symptoms at all – they have no discomfort with the change, so they have no symptoms that need treating. Other women find that herbs or a healthy lifestyle are effective in relieving symptoms. (In Chapter 16 we home in on the herbal route, while in Chapters 18 and 19 we offer lots of information on diet, nutrition, and exercise.) Eating healthily and staying fit go a long way towards keeping your body and mind healthy without the oestrogen they used to rely on.

Sometimes you may need an extra biological boost, which can come in the form of food supplements (calcium, for example) and hormone replacement therapy (HRT).

Because lower levels of oestrogen over prolonged periods of time can result in other medical problems, work with your doctor to find appropriate therapies to prevent these problems.

Menopause Isn't a Disease, So You Don't Need to See a Doctor

Think again! Menopause isn't a medical condition, but that fact doesn't mean you can ignore it. Tell your doctor about any new symptoms you experience or new medical issues that arise as you enter perimenopause and menopause.

Night sweats, fuzzy thinking, interrupted sleep, hot flushes, mood swings, fatigue, and irritability are recognisable (and annoying) symptoms of perimenopause. But these symptoms can also signal more serious medical problems such as anaemia, Epstein–Barr virus, thyroid problems, and other issues. You want to rule out the more serious medical issues before you assume that you're experiencing perimenopause symptoms. So keep track of your symptoms: Write down when, how often, and for how long you experience them, and then share this information with your doctor.

You may think that the main purpose of a visit to your doctor is to *assess* your current health and to *fix* any problems. But as you reach the point in your life at which most women enter perimenopause and menopause, doctors spend a greater amount of time trying to *prevent* the development of serious conditions, including breast cancer, cervical cancer, hypertension, cardiovascular disease, high blood-cholesterol levels, and more.

You Lose the Urge to Have Sex after the Change

Hardly! Nearly half of menopausal women are satisfied with their sex life. If you do your own poll of your premenopausal friends (or tune into a daytime talk show), expect to find that the percentages are pretty comparable. Some women actually find sex more enjoyable – you don't have to worry about getting pregnant, you and your partner have experience under your belts (so you know how to enjoy yourselves and your relationship), and you and your special someone may have more time to spend together without other family members demanding attention.

That said, some women find intercourse painful because of vaginal dryness or vaginal atrophy. If vaginal dryness or atrophy is a problem for you, you can find great remedies at your pharmacy or supermarket or from your doctor. Vaginal moisturisers and vaginal oestrogen pills or creams can treat vaginal dryness. Applying a lubricant during foreplay usually eliminates painful intercourse, too.

Sexual stimulation begets sexual lubrication. In other words, the more you use it, the slower you lose it. Don't forget that 'personal pleasure' can help you stay in shape. In fact, that famous sex doctor, Alfred Kinsey, found that even though marital intercourse declined as women got older, solitary sexual activity didn't decline until women were well past 60. Another study found that even though women's overall lubrication and sexual activity decline *slightly* after menopause, the frequency and pleasure of orgasm does not. For more about the change and your sex life (and making changes to your sex life), check out Chapter 8.

Irregular Vaginal Bleeding Always Means Cancer

Not exactly. Almost all perimenopausal women experience irregular menstrual cycles. In some months, you go 25 days between cycles; in others, you go 38 days. Some months are heavy, and others are light. Or you may even skip a month or two. These menstrual irregularities are generally caused by fluctuating hormones that get out of balance during perimenopause.

If you go through a super-absorbent pad or tampon every couple of hours, experience bleeding after intercourse, or experience bleeding more often than every three weeks, see your doctor to find out what's happening. Sometimes this type of irregular bleeding can signal more serious problems. Also, if you're bleeding between your periods, always consult your doctor.

Humps Accompany Old Age – End of Story

No way! Women don't automatically sprout a dowager's hump as they age. Vertebrae only collapse and result in spinal humps in some cases of *osteoporosis* (brittle bone disease).

If you don't want to acquire a hump, you need to begin strengthening your bones early in life by getting lots of calcium in your diet and exercise in your day. Osteoporosis is largely treatable with medicine and is often preventable with the help of good nutrition, exercise, and calcium substitutes.

If your bones are in bad shape as you approach menopause, several drugs that can slow bone deterioration are on the market. The oestrogen in hormone replacement therapy is also effective at slowing the rate of bone loss. A non-pharmaceutical approach to avoiding a hump is to add regular strength-building exercises to your week.

Only HRT Can Relieve Your Symptoms

False! Although hormone replacement therapy is an effective way to eliminate many annoying menopausal symptoms, you can find alternatives. But remember that less than half of all women experience the symptoms that people associate with menopause (or perimenopause). So you may get lucky and avoid these symptoms without any type of intervention. Also, remember that the symptoms, such as hot flushes, interrupted sleep, fuzzy thinking, mental lapses, and so on, are temporary and eventually go away in their own time.

Now, if these symptoms are making your life miserable, you can try a number of different remedies. Start out by adopting a healthier lifestyle. Here are a few quick ideas (for more info, check out Chapters 18 and 19):

- ✔ Cut down on fats and junk foods.
- ✔ Eat only moderate amounts of meat and protein.
- ✔ Fill your plate with vegetables and fruits.

> ✔ Keep an eye on your alcohol intake. (Don't drink more than three to five units of alcohol a week.)
>
> ✔ Exercise at least three to five days a week for a half-hour each day.

You may also want to try a herbal remedy (such as black cohosh) or include soy in your diet. Edamame (a type of large-seed soybean) and tofu are excellent sources of soy. (For more information on alternative ways to deal with the change, turn to Chapter 16.)

Women Don't Need to Worry about Heart Attacks

Wrong! Heart disease kills many more women each year than cancer. Almost one in two women in the Western world dies of a heart attack or stroke. Oestrogen seems to provide some protection to your cardiovascular system, so women generally have a lower risk of heart attack than men. After menopause, when you no longer produce oestrogen, your risk of heart attack and stroke rises. A healthy diet and regular exercise can help lower your risk of cardiovascular disease.

Most Women Get Really Depressed During Menopause

False! Actually, women tend to get more depressed during the 'procreation' years than during menopause. However, your emotions can take a tumble during perimenopause. Irritability, mood swings, and interrupted sleep can take a toll on your emotions. (For more information on the mental and emotional issues tied to menopause, peruse Chapter 9.) But you can find ways to alleviate these symptoms. A healthy diet and a regular exercise programme help many women alleviate symptoms. Also a slew of pharmaceutical and herbal therapies can help resolve mental and emotional symptoms. (Take a look at Chapters 16 and 17.)

If you fought bouts of depression earlier in life, you may see a return of the symptoms during perimenopause, but remember that perimenopausal symptoms are transient and go away in time. If you experience symptoms or signs of depression, talk to your doctor.

You Break a Bone if You Exercise too Hard

Nope! Weight-bearing exercise (exercise that puts stress on your bones) is one of the best ways to help your body build bone. If you have osteoporosis or your bone density is getting low, the combination of weight-bearing exercise and calcium supplements (with vitamins D and K and magnesium) will prevent further bone loss.

If you normally live a sedentary lifestyle with little or no regular exercise (or you want to change your exercise regime), discuss your exercise plan with a doctor before you begin moving that body. Combining exercises that help your flexibility and balance with a walking programme is a good way to get started. Flexibility and balance exercises can help you avoid falling and fractures. After you have that body moving, try adding weight-bearing exercises to the routine. (Check out Chapter 19 for fantastic fitness suggestions.)

A Blood Test Can Determine whether You're Going through Menopause

Well, here's the deal: Your doctor may test your levels of *follicle stimulating hormone* (FSH) to determine whether you're going through menopause. FSH is the hormone that tells the ovaries to get a follicle ready – this message kicks off your menstrual cycle. As your ovaries slow down, your brain tries to keep things moving at the regular pace, so it shoots out lots of FSH. Also, your brain doesn't see much oestrogen coming back that says, 'Alright already, the follicles are on their way', so FSH keeps on coming. Consistently high levels of FSH indicate the onset of menopause to the medical community.

But here's the catch: FSH levels tell you when your ovaries are pretty close to shutting down follicle production, but they won't tell you if your hormones are in the wild state of fluctuation typical of the perimenopausal years. Unfortunately, most women are most interested in finding out what's going on with their bodies when they just start experiencing weird things like hot flushes, mood swings, and heart palpitations. By the time their FSH levels remain high, they already know the score – periods are pretty much stopped and the test just confirms the logical deduction that menopause is indeed near.

Chapter 21

Meeting More Than Ten Medical Tests for Menopausal Women

. . . .

In This Chapter

▶ Uncovering common medical problems

▶ Having regular gynaecological check-ups

▶ Relying on early detection of disease

. . . .

*I*n this chapter we list some of the basic health tests that help your doctor identify diseases and other problems in their early stages – when they're more easily treatable. This topic's so important that we talk about more than ten tests – which goes against the letter, but not the spirit, of the Part of Tens law. *Early detection* is the key to successful treatment of nearly every disease that affects menopausal women. Avoiding the tests doesn't mean that you can avoid the related diseases, so visit your doctor regularly and follow through with his or her recommendations.

Pelvic Examination and Cervical Smear

No one likes opening their legs and having their genitals examined, but doing so helps you avoid nasty problems down the line. Ideally, you should have an annual gynaecological screen – even if you have to pay for it privately, although some women are lucky enough to receive an annual medical as a perk of their job. The National Health Service (NHS) normally provides only three-yearly cervical smears unless your doctor detects abnormalities that need more frequent follow-up. During a gynaecological examination, your doctor checks your female organs, including your breasts, vaginal tissue, cervix, and uterus. Your doctor also performs a *cervical smear* to test for cervical cancer.

If you've had a complete hysterectomy and removal of your ovaries for benign reasons, ideally you should still have a breast and pelvic exam every year. If the body of your uterus is removed but your cervix is left in place (sub-total hysterectomy), you still need regular cervical smears too.

Rectal Examination

Most people squirm when this exam is the subject at hand, but the risks of postponing a rectal exam are quite devastating to you and your loved ones. Regular rectal exams can help detect problems early – when your doctor can treat them more easily and painlessly. Part of this test is a *digital exam*, in which your doctor checks your organs for signs of disease. The doctor inserts a gloved finger into your rectum to evaluate the health of your tissues. Keep in mind that the long-term benefits greatly outweigh the short-term unpleasantness of the procedure. And also remember that your doctor *chose* this field of medicine.

The other part of this exam is a *faecal occult blood test*, which lets your doctor check whether you have blood in your stool. The presence of blood is an indication of problems, such as cancer, in your colon.

Ideally you should have a rectal exam once a year during your annual medical check-up, especially after the age of 50. The NHS bowel cancer screening programme aims to offer faecal occult blood screening every two years to all people in the UK between the ages of 60 and 69 years. People over 70 can also request screening kits.

Colonoscopy

If your faecal occult blood test is positive, your doctor will arrange a colonoscopy to look for a possible colon cancer.

Colon cancer is the second most common cancer affecting women, after breast cancer. No one likes the thought of a colonoscopy test, and women often avoid discussing the issue until they have symptoms. The problem is that people very often don't experience any symptoms until colon cancer is in an advanced stage – a point when successful treatment is much more difficult. But colon cancer progresses very slowly and is readily treatable if caught early, which is why this test is so important.

During a colonoscopy, your doctor can find and remove precancerous polyps (doctors know them as *adenomatous polyps*) before they have a chance to turn into cancer. The night before your colonoscopy, you drink a potion that helps to clean out your colon. You have a light sedative, and your doctor inserts a flexible scope into your colon to view your colon walls in search of polyps or other unhealthy tissue. If your doctor finds a polyp, he or she can remove it and send it to a laboratory for analysis. Lab analysis determines whether the polyp is benign or precancerous.

After a positive faecal occult blood test, about 5 in 10 people undergoing a colonoscopy receive a normal result, 4 in 10 are found to have a polyp (which is removed), and about 1 in 10 are found to have a colon cancer.

Bone-Density Screening

If you can, have at least one bone-density screening before you're menopausal. If your family (sister, mother, or grandmother) has a history of osteoporosis, your doctor is usually happy to arrange this test for you, ideally when you're in your late thirties. If you've never had a bone screening and you're over 40, talk to your doctor about your options and consider paying for the test privately when you're around 40 to get a baseline bone-density screening. The results provide your doctor with something to compare future screenings with. If you show signs of bone loss in this or subsequent tests, your doctor may suggest that you have bone screenings every two years.

Mammogram

Early detection is the key to reducing your risk of breast cancer. The NHS breast screening programme is available for all women aged 50 and over. Those aged 50–70 years are automatically invited for mammography every three years. Those aged 70 or older can make an appointment without an invitation. Some experts recommend getting annual mammograms from the age of 40 years, but this practice remains controversial. The reason that NHS screening starts at 50 is because most breast cancers occur in postmenopausal women, and because the breast tissue of younger women is more dense, making interpretation of mammograms more difficult. If you have a family history of breast cancer at an early age, however, you are entitled to mammography before the age of 50 years. In such cases, you and your doctor decide between you the age at which you enter the breast screening programme.

Cholesterol Screening

A cholesterol screening checks your total cholesterol, *LDL cholesterol* (bad cholesterol), *HDL cholesterol* (good cholesterol), and *triglycerides* (another form of fat found in your blood) and computes your cholesterol ratio. Take this simple blood test every five years. Your doctor takes a blood test first thing in the morning when you're still fasting – so nothing to eat or drink for 12 hours before the test. If your doctor identifies problems with your cholesterol or triglyceride levels or you have a history of high blood pressure, diabetes, thyroid problems, or obesity, your doctor may want to screen you more frequently.

Fasting Blood-Glucose Test

Adult-onset diabetes can lead to coronary heart disease, so you want to diagnose this problem early. Ideally, you should start having your blood sugar (*glucose*) tested (or at least a urine dipstick test for glucose) when you're 20 and repeat the test every three to five years – more frequently if you experience problems. The blood-glucose test is a simple blood test administered after you've had nothing to eat or drink for 12 hours (that's where the *fasting* part of the name comes from). Your doctor can also screen you for diabetes by checking for sugar in your urine.

Thyroid Screening

The symptoms of thyroid problems and the symptoms of menopause are often quite similar. If you feel tired all the time, feel the cold and are tending to put on weight, ask your doctor for a thyroid screening test. The screening measures your levels of thyroid stimulating hormone (TSH) and thyroid antibodies. See *Thyroid for Dummies* by Dr Sarah Brewer and Dr Alan Rubin (Wiley).

CA125 Test

Doctors don't routinely perform this blood test but it's worth asking your doctor about it if you have a family history of ovarian cancer or if you're having abdominal bloating or pain or other symptoms that evade diagnosis or don't respond to other treatments. Levels of the CA125 antigen often rise with the presence of ovarian cancer, endometriosis, ovarian cysts, fibroids, and even the early stages of pregnancy.

The CA125 test isn't considered diagnostic for ovarian cancer because higher levels of CA125 don't necessarily indicate ovarian cancer, and sometimes, levels don't rise if you have ovarian cancer. But high levels of CA125 are sometimes an early warning of ovarian cancer and so, if you have high levels, your doctor should pursue additional tests until ovarian cancer is ruled out.

Ovarian Hormone Screening

Out of necessity, the standard practice for prescribing hormone therapy is a method of trial and error – a 'try this regimen and let me know how you feel' kind of approach. Everybody processes hormones differently, so the amount of hormone in a medication isn't the amount that reaches your bloodstream. For example, the same form of oestrogen may affect two women differently. And your body may respond better to some oestrogens than others.

The key to what works and what doesn't is the amount of *oestradiol* (the active form of oestrogen) that your body produces in response to the oestrogen you're taking. The only accurate way to know how much oestradiol you're churning out is to draw blood and analyse it for hormone levels. (Saliva tests are available, but they're less accurate.)

That said, the majority of doctors stick with the standard dosing formulas and do the trial-and-error thing until you tell them that you're feeling better. An alternative (ovarian hormone screening) is available, however, and is a bit more objective. Oestradiol levels that are persistently below 300 picomol/litre (pmol/L) result in the typical hot flushes, interrupted sleep, mood swings, and other annoying perimenopausal symptoms. If your levels drop much below 300 picomol/litre, you risk suffering from bone loss and cardiovascular issues. So the key is to maintain your oestradiol levels between 300 pmol/L and 500 pmol/L.

If your doctor is experimenting with hormone replacement therapy he or she may check your current hormone levels to see how effectively your therapy is working.

Stress Test

You may think that your life is one big stress test, but actually, a stress test is a legitimate medical procedure. A stress test is basically an electrocardiogram (ECG) that a technician performs while you walk on a treadmill. You may have an ECG in your youth for example, when taking out life insurance or as part of an annual medical. The purpose of the exercise stress test is to see how your heart responds to the effects of exercise. If you're overweight, have high blood pressure, or experience chest pain or shortness of breath with mild exertion, your doctor may suggest a stress test. Your doctor may also perform a stress test to check out your heart before you begin a new exercise programme.

The procedure is simple. A technician sticks electrical wires on your chest to record the electrical activity in your heart. This information tells the doctor if your heart is getting enough oxygen or is showing signs of damage. To stress your heart, you walk on a special treadmill while you're plugged into the ECG.

You also get a stress test if your doctor suspects that you have coronary heart disease; otherwise, if you have private medical insurance, it's a good idea to ask about having a baseline reading at 40 and then take the test every three to five years. The risk of heart attack rises after menopause, so don't overlook the importance of checking out the health of your heart.

Chapter 22

Running Through Ten Terrific Fitness Programmes for Menopausal Women

. . . .

In This Chapter

▶ Finding your flexibility

▶ Stretching for strength

▶ Coordinating cardiac training

. . . .

*N*eed help getting your fitness programme off the ground? In this chapter, we offer lots of good suggestions to help you clear the runway.

Many women dread the thought of a workout because, to them, the concept implies sweat (sadly, ladies don't just glow), finding time they don't have, and too much effort. If this description fits you, think again. You can find a workout that fits your schedule and desired level of energy output. And if you hate to sweat, check out the water-based workouts in this chapter.

Always warm up and cool down for five to ten minutes before and after you workout. If you have trouble with your heart, blood pressure, cholesterol, or diabetes, if you suffer from a respiratory condition, if you're overweight, if you smoke, or if you are, in all honesty, a couch potato, discuss your physical fitness plans with your doctor before you get started. Try to think of your weekly fitness routine as a buffet: Include a little of everything on your plate – aerobic training, strength training, flexibility, and balance-building exercises.

Core-Stability Training

Core-stability training is a great way to improve your balance and flexibility, reduce your risk of injury, and lessen the amount of soreness you get with performing daily activities. Core stability training is basically strength training that targets the muscle groups making up the core of your body – your abdominal, lower back, hip, and pelvic muscles are the primary focus. Strengthening your core muscles allows them to do their job (maintaining your body's stability and balance) better.

These muscles are the foundation of support for just about any activity your body does. The every-day aches and pains that many women feel are often the result of weakened core-muscle groups. Your body tries to compensate for these weak muscles, which can lead to pain in your lower back and arm and leg joints.

Here's how core-stability training works: You incorporate exercises that challenge your abdominal, lower-back, hip, pelvic, and oblique muscles. You can strengthen these muscles with traditional exercises and callisthenic-type movements. (Chapter 19 is full of effective exercises to help you strengthen these muscles, and you will find even more in the books included in the resources in Appendix B.)

Additional toys are available that can add variety and fun to your workout and make your workout more effective. Equipment such as balance balls, stability boards, and old-fashioned medicine balls makes targeting the muscles that help maintain your stability and balance easier. Strengthening these muscles can also improve your posture.

Cycling

Perhaps walking and running are too slow for you, and you're not really a water person. Taking up cycling, whether in the gym or on the road, is another good option, providing a cardio workout. Cycling provides a great aerobic workout that improves your cardiovascular health, muscle tone, and stamina.

If you're just getting started, you may want to try a stationary bike at your local gym or health club. Try riding for six minutes at 15 miles per hour (or 55 revolutions per minute), five times a week. Gradually work up to 20 to 25 minutes, five times a week, at the same speed. As you get accustomed to cycling, you can build up your aerobic fitness even more by increasing your speed.

After spending time in the saddle, you may want to try a spinning class. A *spinning class* is a group indoor-cycling class that really helps build your aerobic fitness. You can find spinning classes at many local sports centres, community colleges, and health clubs across the country. An instructor guides each class and makes your 'ride' on a special stationary bike as challenging as you like.

If you're more of the outdoor type, get your bike out the garage, check the brakes and tyres, and go for a ride. Don't forget about safety: Always wear a helmet and choose a route in a safe area that has little traffic and contains few hills (to start with at least!).

Start by riding for ten minutes, five times a week. Add two minutes to your workout each week (riding five times a week) so that by the end of Week 11 you're riding for 30 minutes five times a week.

Elliptical Training

The elliptical-training machine is a relatively new but terrific way to get aerobic, cardio exercise without hurting your joints with high-impact workouts. An elliptical trainer looks like a combination of a treadmill and a climber that grew arms! The machine is called an elliptical trainer because your feet move in the shape of an oval during the workout instead of back and forth like they do on a treadmill, or up and down like they move on a climber. Because your feet follow an oval path, the exercise is low impact but still provides a full range of motion for your legs. The arms on the machine go back and forth while you stride, so that you get a total body workout.

Pilates

Even though Pilates (pronounced puh-*lah*-teez) is a fairly recent form of exercise, its roots date back to the 1920s. Think of Pilates as a combination of yoga, stretching, and callisthenics, all rolled up into one set of exercises.

These exercises work on many of the same muscle groups as a core-stability training programme (check out 'Core-Stability Training' earlier in this chapter) and offer many of the same advantages. In Pilates, you perform slow, extremely focused movements that work the muscles in your abdomen, lower back, and buttocks. And yes, For Dummies has a snazzy yellow-and-black covered book on this subject too – *Pilates For Dummies* by Ellie Herman (Wiley).

Running

Running reduces your risk of developing heart disease, high blood pressure, adult-onset diabetes, and several types of cancer. It also increases the levels of good (HDL) cholesterol in your blood, which helps you to get rid of the bad (LDL) cholesterol. (For more information on cholesterol levels, see Chapter 5.) Running also improves your cardiovascular and respiratory systems and can help you to control your weight. (Some people lose up to 5.4 kilograms (12 pounds) the first year they start running without reducing the calories they eat.)

Getting started on a running regimen is easy: Just chart out a course (in a safe area) and get a pair of good running shoes. If you're a beginner, try running a mile. If you can't do a mile, try alternating between running and walking until you can cover the entire mile without the walking part. Then add a little distance at a time. Initially schedule about 30 minutes of running time and build up the duration as you go.

If you have joint or back problems, running may not suit you in which case walk as briskly as you can, on even ground, for a good, aerobic workout, instead.

Swimming

Swimming is easy on your joints and helps to build muscle strength equally on both sides of your body. In fact, swimming forces you to use all your muscles. Now that's what we call a workout! Swimming is a great exercise for people looking to increase their overall physical fitness or to recover from an injury.

If you've had a hip or knee replaced or you suffer from arthritis, swimming is an excellent way to maintain aerobic conditioning through low-impact exercise.

T'ai Chi

T'ai chi helps to stretch and tone your muscles, relieve stress, and improve balance and circulation. You may even find that your blood pressure is lower. This ancient, Chinese form of exercise, meditation, and self-defence involves controlled movements done slowly and continuously. The forms are similar to those used in other martial arts. If t'ai chi sounds like it may be just up your alley, *T'ai Chi For Dummies* by Therese Iknoian with Manny Fuentes (Wiley) is a great place to start.

Walking

Walking is a free and convenient way to relieve stress, improve your fitness, build muscle tone and strengthen both your heart and your bones. To make sure that your efforts bring you good health:

- ✔ Walk for at least 30 minutes per session.
- ✔ Walk at least four times a week.
- ✔ Walk at a moderately intense pace. You should cover about 3½ miles in an hour (or 1¾ miles in half an hour).

Refer to Chapter 19, which has a whole section on how to design a walking programme.

Water Aerobics

Here's a great cardio exercise if you feel out of place jumping around in an aerobics class in front of a bunch of other people. In water aerobics your legs are under water, so if you miss a step or have to take a breather, no one else notices. Water aerobics helps you work your cardiovascular system, arm muscles, and leg muscles. The exercise is less stressful on your joints than many exercise programmes, and it improves your balance and coordination. Many health clubs and public swimming pools offer classes with professional trainers. Water aerobics is a great way to have fun, stay cool, and get active.

Yoga

Yoga is a great way to improve your health. Studies show that yoga reduces stress, lowers blood pressure, relieves arthritis, and builds strength and flexibility. The breathing techniques used during a yoga workout help increase the oxygen levels in your blood.

Some styles of yoga focus more on the spiritual aspects, such as meditation and chanting, and are great for stress reduction and relaxation. Other forms focus on body alignment and challenging workouts that improve muscle tone, balance, and flexibility. All forms of yoga use poses and breathing techniques to heighten the mind–body connection. Check out *Yoga For Dummies* by Georg Fauerstein and Larry Payne (Wiley) for more information.

Part VI
Appendixes

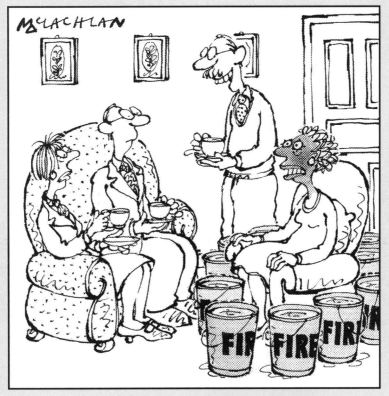

'Poor Dorothy's going through the
menopause – terrible hot flushes.'

In this part . . .

Literature on menopause is often filled with a dazzling array of medical terms, jargon, and other overstuffed phrases. We, of course, try to simplify this state of affairs. But, in case you run across a word that you need a quick definition for, whether it's in this book or other literature about menopause, we include a glossary of terms – Appendix A. In Appendix B, we provide you with a bunch of additional sources of information – from books to Web sites – that do a great job covering menopause and other health-related issues of interest to women.

Appendix A

Glossary

Adenomatous polyp: Precancerous polyp in the lining of the colon.

Amenorrhoea: Condition in women who haven't gone through *menopause* in which they miss menstrual periods for several months in a row.

Androgens: Hormones that produce masculine effects on the body such as a deep voice and facial hair. Both men and women produce androgens, although women produce them in much smaller amounts.

Angina: Pain in the chest, arm, or neck due to lack of blood flow to the heart. Angina is usually a symptom of *coronary heart disease.*

Antioxidant: A substance, such as vitamins A, C, and E, and beta-carotene, that protects cells from damaging *oxidation.* Antioxidants help to protect against premature ageing and certain diseases.

Atherosclerosis: Hardening and furring up of the arteries due to a build-up of *cholesterol* and other substances in the walls of blood vessels. This process causes a narrowing of the blood vessels and can lead to *coronary heart disease*.

Atrophy: See *vaginal atrophy*.

Bisphosphonates: A group of medications used to treat *osteoporosis* that stimulate bone growth and slow down bone destruction.

Body mass index (BMI): A method of estimating body fat using a weight-to-height ratio. For weight in pounds and height in inches, BMI = weight/height^2.

Carcinoma *in situ:* Condition in which abnormal cancer cells are located in a confined space and haven't spread to other areas. At this stage, most cancers are successfully treatable.

Cardiovascular disease (CVD): Disease that affects the heart, arteries, veins, and capillaries.

Cholesterol: A fat-like substance that comprises an important part of the body's cells. Three main forms of cholesterol are found in blood: high-density lipids (*HDL*), low-density lipids (*LDL*), and very-low-density lipids (VLDL). Found in animal-derived foods.

Combination therapy: A type of *hormone replacement therapy* in which a woman takes an oestrogen and a *progestogen.*

Conjugated oestrogens: A mixture of oestrogens sometimes used in *hormone replacement therapy.* They're chemically different from human *oestrogen* and can come from either plants or horses.

Continuous combination therapy: A type of hormone therapy regime in which a woman takes an *oestrogen* and *progestogen* together throughout the month.

Coronary heart disease (CHD): A disease in which the blood vessels that supply the heart become narrow and restrict the flow of oxygenated blood to the heart. *Atherosclerosis* is the process that leads to coronary heart disease.

Corpus luteum: A yellow sac formed from the remains of the *egg follicle* after the egg releases. The corpus luteum produces *progesterone.*

Cyclic combination therapy: A type of hormone therapy regime in which a woman takes oestrogen by itself for several days of the month, followed by a period in which she takes both *oestrogen* and *progestogen.*

Deep-vein thrombosis (DVT): Blood clots in the veins running deep through the body (usually in the upper arm, calf, thigh, or pelvic areas). These veins lie deeper under the skin than surface veins and return more blood to the heart. A clot in one of these veins causes more complications than a clot in surface veins, such as a *pulmonary embolism*.

DEXA: Abbreviation for *dual-energy x-ray absorptiometry* – a method of measuring bone-mineral density. Used to screen for *osteoporosis.*

DHEA: Abbreviation for *dehydroepiandrosterone,* which is a male hormone produced in a woman's adrenal glands and *ovaries.*

Dowager's hump: An old term for an apparent hump in the back of some people with osteoporosis. Caused by the collapse of vertebrae in the spine due to porous (brittle) bone. The term comes from the outdated idea that osteoporosis is a condition that strikes only postmenopausal women (little old ladies, or dowagers).

Endometrium: The lining of the uterus.

Fibrinogen: A type of protein that helps blood to clot.

Follicle: A little sac created from an *oocyte* (egg seed) in the ovary. The follicle produces *oestrogen* in the ovary. At least one of these little guys usually releases an egg each month during a woman's reproductive years. After the egg is released, the follicle collapses to form a *corpus luteum.*

Follicle-stimulating hormone (FSH): A hormone produced in the brain that triggers the *ovaries* to begin developing *follicles.* Doctors consider continued high levels of FSH are an indication of *menopause.* The FSH keeps trying to stimulate follicle production when the cupboard is bare – the ovary can no longer crank out follicles – which is a sign that the ovary is entering retirement and you're entering menopause.

HDL: Abbreviation for high-density lipoprotein. HDL is 'good cholesterol' because it carries fat from body cells back to the liver for excretion so that it doesn't hang around in the circulation to encourage *atherosclerosis. Lipoproteins* are made up of protein and fat. Lipoproteins with more protein than fat are called high-density lipids; a lipoprotein with more fat than protein is called a low-density lipoprotein *(LDL).*

Hormone: Chemicals produced in one part of the body and which travel to activate functions in other parts of the body.

Hormone-receptor site: A 'docking station' for hormones on a cell where hormones can connect to cells to manipulate them.

Hormone replacement therapy (HRT): Treatment designed to adjust hormone levels using synthetic or natural female hormones. Doctors generally administer this treatment to women going through *perimenopause* and/or *menopause.*

Hypertension: Medical term for high blood pressure.

Hysterectomy: Surgical removal of the uterus. A *total* hysterectomy removes only the uterus. A *sub-total* hysterectomy removes the body of the uterus but leaves behind the cervix. A *total* hysterectomy plus bilateral salpingo-oophorectomy (BSO) removes the uterus, fallopian tubes and the *ovaries.* Removal of the ovaries causes *surgical menopause.*

Incontinence: See *Urinary incontinence*.

Interstitial cystitis (IC): A bladder condition that's hard to diagnose, but the symptoms include mild discomfort, pressure, tenderness, or intense pain in the bladder and surrounding pelvic area. Symptoms may include an urgent need to urinate (*urgency*), a frequent need to urinate (*frequency*), or a combination of these symptoms. Researchers don't know the causes of IC, and few treatments are effective.

Isoflavone: See *phytooestrogen.*

Labia: The lips of the vaginal opening. **See also** *vulva.*

LDL: Abbreviation for low-density lipoprotein – or 'bad cholesterol'. LDLs are found in the bloodstream and are thought to carry cholesterol from the liver to body cells. Eating a diet high in saturated fats and cholesterol will raise your LDL levels. The higher the LDL level, the greater the incidence of *coronary heart disease*.

Libido: Sex drive.

Lobules: Milk-producing glands in the breast. Cancer sometimes starts in the lobules.

Luteinising hormone (LH): A hormone made in the pituitary gland. In women, it triggers *ovulation.*

Menarche: The onset of menstrual periods, which signals the beginning of a woman's reproductive maturation at puberty.

Menopause: The technical meaning is the end of menstruation – no *menses* for 12 months. Because periods are so irregular in the months leading up to menopause, the medical community generally doesn't consider you to be officially menopausal until 12 months after your last period. The media uses this term pretty loosely to refer to all stages of menopause including *perimenopause,* menopause, and *postmenopause.* In this book we restrict usage of the term 'perimenopause' to the stage after a woman is officially menopausal.

Menses: The periodic flow of blood from the uterus – your period. The word derives from the Latin word for *month.*

Oestradiol: The active form of *oestrogen* made in the *ovaries* prior to *menopause*. The most potent form of oestrogen in humans. Plays a role in many bodily functions.

Oestriol: Form of *oestrogen* only produced during pregnancy.

Oestrogen: A female hormone produced in the *ovaries* and in the adrenal glands.

Oestrogen receptor: A 'docking station' on a cell that allows that particular body part to make use of *oestrogen*. Oestrogen receptors are located all over a woman's body but are highly concentrated in oestrogen-sensitive tissues such as bone, uterus and breast tissue.

Oestrone: A type of *oestrogen* made by the *ovaries,* adrenal glands, and body fat before *menopause.* After menopause, body fat makes oestrone; therefore, oestrone is the only type of oestrogen in good supply after menopause. Oestrone is less active than *oestradiol* oestrogen.

Osteoblast: Cells that build new bone.

Osteoclast: Cells that break down bone during the bone-maintenance process.

Osteopenia: Loss of bone density that isn't sufficiently severe to diagnose *osteoporosis.* If action isn't taken to better maintain the bone, this condition will turn into osteoporosis over time.

Osteoporosis: Loss of bone density. Makes bones brittle, porous, and weak.

Ovaries: Female sex organs that store egg 'seeds' (*oocytes*), some of which develop into *follicles.* You're born with two ovaries. They produce the hormones *oestrogen* and *progesterone* as well as a small amount of *testosterone.*

Ovulation: The process in which an egg is released from the *follicle.*

Oxidation: Technically, this term refers to the process through which oxygen combines with another substance – like when metal turns to rust. So what does this have to do with menopause? Unstable oxygen molecules, *free radicals* in med speak, are produced as your body cells go about their daily chores. Because they're unstable, free radicals react with other molecules as they move through your body. Oxidation does some good things, but it also damages healthy cells, which can lead to cancer, heart disease, and other ailments common to menopausal women – including wrinkles.

Palpitation: A fluttering sensation that you may experience in your chest, accompanied by a rapid heartbeat.

Perimenopause: Time frame before *menopause* when hormones fluctuate radically, periods are often irregular, and women may experience physical and emotional symptoms (such as hot flushes, heart palpitations, mood swings, irritability, and crying spells). Perimenopause may begin ten years prior to menopause but more typically begins four to six years prior to menopause and continues through the first year after menstrual periods stop.

Phytooestrogen: *Oestrogen* produced by plants (such as the soybean plant) that binds with human *oestrogen receptors* and results in weak, oestrogen-like actions. *Isoflavones* are one form of phytooestrogen.

Polyp: A non-cancerous growth that protrudes from tissues. This book discusses *adenomatous polyps* of the colon.

Postmenopause: The years after *menopause* when the ovaries are no longer functioning. This is the time when health conditions associated with long periods of low *oestrogen* (*osteoporosis* and *cardiovascular disease*) are your top concern.

Premature menopause: Experiencing menopause at an unusually early age (like in your thirties). Premature menopause leaves you at risk of osteoporosis and higher cholesterol fairly early in life.

Premenopausal: Term associated with women who haven't yet gone through *menopause.*

Progesterone: A female hormone produced by the *ovaries* after *ovulation* to prepare the uterus for fertilisation.

Progestogen: Synthetic form of the natural hormone *progesterone.*

Pulmonary embolism: Blockage of an artery in the lungs by a blood clot. Pulmonary embolism can result from a *deep-vein thrombosis*.

Sequential combination therapy: A type of hormone therapy regime in which a woman takes oestrogen, followed by progestogen, followed by a period in which no hormones are taken.

SERMs: Abbreviation for *selective oestrogen receptor modulators* – special 'designer hormones' used in *hormone therapy.* (Oestrogen is spelled 'estrogen' in the US, which is why this class of drug is known as SERMs, not SORMs.) SERMs can activate *oestrogen receptors* in some parts of the body while blocking oestrogen receptors in other parts of the body. SERMs are particularly useful as they provide the bone benefits of HRT without increasing the risk of breast cancer.

Serotonin: A brain chemical that regulates sleep, mood, *libido,* pain, and more.

Surgical menopause: *Menopause* that results from the surgical removal of the ovaries.

Testosterone: A male hormone produced by the *ovaries* in low levels. Helps to maintain muscle mass, bone, and *libido* in women.

Transdermal: A method of delivering medication in which the medication is absorbed through the skin and goes directly into the bloodstream.

Triglyceride: The chemical form of fats circulating in the bloodstream and which act as building blocks for making *cholesterol.*

Unopposed oestrogen: A type of hormone therapy regime in which a woman uses *oestrogen* without a *progestogen* to balance it.

Urethra: The little canal through which you urinate.

Urinary incontinence: The inability to keep from urinating.

Urinary-tract infection (UTI): An infection that affects the bladder, *urethra,* or kidneys.

Vaginal atrophy: Thinning and drying of vaginal tissue often occurring during *perimenopause* and *menopause.*

Vulva: Collective term for the external female genital organs, consisting of the *mons* (fleshy, rounded area covered by pubic hair), *labia* (lips or folds of the vagina), *hymen* (thin mucous membrane that keeps the vagina partially closed), *clitoris* (a woman's pleasure spot), and some glands.

Appendix B

Resources

· ·

*I*f you're interested in finding more information about menopause, hormones, and related conditions, here's a quick guide to some terrific resources.

Brilliant Books about Menopause, Health, Fitness, and Related Issues

The following are some excellent reference books. They contain lots of good information and the authors wrote them with the layperson in mind. You can find these books at your local library or bookstore.

Getting Stronger: Weight Training for Men and Women (Revised Edition) by Bill Pearl (Shelter Publications). Many women really don't know where to start when they're first told to incorporate weight-bearing exercise into their workout. If you're a bit perplexed about the subject, pick up this title. You can find out what to look for in a health club, how to use different types of weight machines, how to condition specific muscles, and how to create a workout programme to get in shape for your favourite sport. Nice illustrations accompany all exercise descriptions and show you exactly what to do and what muscle you'll work.

Weight Training For Dummies by Liz Neporent, Suzanne Schlosberg, and Shirley Archer (Wiley). The *For Dummies* take on weight training – what more could you need? Featuring illustrated step-by-step exercises plus tips on equipment and specialised workouts, this friendly guide shows you how to get started and get results – at home or at the gym, using free weights or weight machines.

Healthy Women, Healthy Lives by Susan E. Hankinson, Graham A. Colditz, JoAnn E. Manson, and Frank E. Speizer (Simon & Schuster). With that many authors, it has to be good. This book offers important lessons about reducing your risk for many chronic diseases and several forms of cancer. Using results from one of the largest studies of women in the world, the Nurses' Health Study, this resource can help you make better-informed personal-health choices. It's informative and yet very easy to read and understand.

Intimate Relations: Living and Loving in Later Life by Dr Sarah Brewer (Age Concern). A rewarding sex life is an important part of wellbeing and a loving relationship at all stages of adult life. Menopause can bring a number of sexual challenges, but this book helps you to maintain loving, intimate relationships through menopause and beyond.

Is It Me, Or Is It Hot In Here? A Modern Woman's Guide to the Menopause by Jenni Murray (Ebury Press (UK)). Compulsory reading for women needing help and advice on the complexities of the menopause, and for the men who are trying to understand them.

Matt Roberts' Fat Loss Plan (Dorling Kindersley). This book is a fabulous source of exercise and healthy eating information. It offers day-by-day personalised plans to help you eat right, lose weight and gain a fitter body; and you don't have to go anywhere near a gym or give up your life. Well illustrated and inspiring!

Menopause: The Complete Guide to Maintaining Health and Well-being and Managing Your Life by Dr Miriam Stoppard (Dorling Kindersley). Does what it says on the tin! Helps every woman feel her best throughout this crucial time and in the years beyond. Excellent information on symptoms, HRT, complementary approaches, nutrition, exercise and maintaining a healthy, active sex life.

The New Natural Alternatives to HRT by Marilyn Glenville (Kyle Cathie). This book provides lots of information on nutritional and other natural approaches to menopause. Interestingly, this author has concerns about the use of isoflavones as well as the use of HRT.

Relate Guide to Sex in Loving Relationships by Sarah Litvinoff (Vermilion). This book aims to help you turn a disappointing sex life into an enjoyable and fulfilling one.

Screaming to be Heard: Hormone Connections Women Suspect and Doctors Still Ignore by Elizabeth Lee Vliet (M. Evans and Company). This book is a terrific resource if you want to know how your natural hormones work and how menopause changes things. The title reflects the author's indignation at the lack of solid research and medical training in the field of hormone therapy. Vliet draws upon her medical experience and uses scenarios and cases from her professional encounters.

Stretching by Bob Anderson (Shelter Publications). This book is celebrating its 20th anniversary, and it's still the bible on the subject of stretching. The updates include new stretches for inline skating and rock climbing (not so popular 20 years ago), but the title stays faithful to its original principle that people of all ages and abilities need to stay flexible and fit to keep well. If you're currently a couch potato, start with this book. It contains stretches that take you from square one and prepare you for an exercise programme. For the more-active woman, *Stretching* offers treasures that can help you push your sport or exercise performance to the next level.

The Aerobics Program for Total Well Being: Exercise/Diet/Emotional Balance by Kenneth H. Cooper (Bantam Doubleday Dell). Okay, this book was first introduced in 1985, but it still works. If you only get one book about maintaining your wellbeing, get this one. Whether you're just getting started or you have 20 marathons under your belt, you'll take something away from reading this book. Exercise, diet, and emotional balance are key to keeping your cardiovascular system and bones healthy – just the parts that trouble menopausal women.

The Seven Ages of Woman: A lifetime guide to feeling good, by Dr Rosemary Leonard (Transworld Publishers Ltd (UK)). This book covers menopause and a whole range of other mental and physical issues you may face throughout your lifetime.

Cracking Contact Details for Women

In this section we list some organisations that can provide further help and advice concerning the menopause. If you have access to the Internet, the world of health and nutrition is at your fingertips. We list some excellent Web sites that provide information and can link you to other good sites.

Cancer

Breakthrough Breast Cancer 246 High Holborn, London, WC1V 7EX; Helpline: 08080 100 200; Web site: www.breakthrough.org.uk

Breast Cancer Care Kiln House, 210 New Kings Road, London SW6 4NZ; Helpline: 0808 800 6000; Web site: www.breastcancercare.org.uk

Cancerbackup 3 Bath Place, Rivington Street, London EC2A 3JR; Helpline: 0808 800 1234; Web site: www.cancerbackup.org.uk

Cancer Research UK PO Box 123 Lincoln's Inn Fields, London, WC2A 3PX; Phone: 020 7121 6699; Web site: www.cancerresearchuk.org

NHS Breast Screening Programme NHS Cancer Screening Programmes, Don Valley House, Savile Street East, Sheffield S4 7UQ; Phone: 0114 271 1060; Web site: www.cancerscreening.nhs.uk/breastscreen

Complementary medicine

British Complementary Medicine Association PO Box 5122, Bournemouth, Dorset BH8 0WG; Phone: 0845 345 5977; Web site: www.bcma.co.uk

British Holistic Medical Association PO Box 371, Bridgwater, Somerset TA6 9BG; Phone: 01278 722000; Web site: www.bhma.org

British Homeopathic Association, Hahnemann House, 29 Park Street West, Luton, Bedfordshire LU1 3BE; Phone: 0870 444 3950; Web site: www.trusthomeopathy.org

Complementary Medical Association Web site: www.the-cma.org.uk

General Council and Register of Naturopaths Goswell House, 2 Goswell Road, Street, Avon BA16 0JG; Phone: 08707 456984; Web site: www.naturopathy.org.uk

Institute for Complementary Medicine PO Box 194, London SE16 7QZ; Phone: 020 7237 5165; Web site: www.i-c-m.org.uk

International Federation of Professional Aromatherapists 82 Ashby Road, Hinckley, Leicestershire LE10 1SN; Phone: 01455 637987; Web site www.ifparoma.org

National Institute of Medical Herbalists Elm House, 54 Mary Arches Street, Exeter EX4 3BA; Phone: 01392 426022; Web site: www.nimh.org.uk

Cardiovascular disease

Blood Pressure Association, 60 Cranmer Terrace, London SW17 0QS; Phone: 020 8772 4994; Web site: www.bpassoc.org.uk

British Heart Foundation 14 Fitzhardinge Street, London W1H 6DH; Phone: 020 7935 0185; Heart Information Line: 08450 70 80 70; Web site: www.bhf.org.uk

British Hypertension Society Clinical Sciences Building, Level 5, Leicester Royal Infirmary, PO Box 65, Leicester LE2 7LX; Phone: 07717 467 973; Web site: www.bhsoc.org

Menopause

Menopause Amarant Trust 80 Lambeth Road, London SE1 7PW; Helpline: 01293 413000; Web site: www.amarantmenopausetrust.org.uk

Menopause Matters Web site: www.menopausematters.co.uk

Natural Menopause Advice Service PO Box 71, Leatherhead, Surrey KT22 7DP; Web site: www.nmas.org.uk

Women's Health Concern Whitehall House, 41 Whitehall, London SW1A 2BY; Helpline: 0845 123 2319; Web site: www.womens-health-concern.org

Nutrition

British Association for Nutritional Therapy BANT, 27 Old Gloucester Street, London WC1N 3XX; Phone: 0870 6061284; Web site: www.bant.org.uk

British Dietetic Association Private Practice, 5th Floor, Charles House, 148/9 Great Charles Street, Queensway, Birmingham B3 3HT; Phone: 0121 200 8080; Web site: www.bda.uk.com

Dietitians Unlimited Freelance Dietitians Group, 22 Birkbeck Road, North Finchley, London; Web site: www.dietitiansunlimited.co.uk

Natural Health Advisory Service PO Box 268, Lewes, East Sussex BN7 1QN; Phone: 01273 609699; Web site: www.naturalhealthas.com

The Nutrition Society 10 Cambridge Court, 210 Shepherds Bush Road, London W6 7NJ; Phone: 020 7602 0228; Web site: www.nutritionsociety.org.uk

Osteoporosis

National Osteoporosis Society Camerton, Bath BA2 0PJ; Helpline: 0845 450 0230; Web site: www.nos.org.uk

Relationship counselling

Relate Phone: 0845 456 1310; Web site: www.relate.org.uk Phone or use the Web site to find your local Relate office.

Women's health

BBC Women's Health www.bbc.co.uk/health/womens_health

Natural Health Website for Women www.marilynglenville.com

NetDoctor www.netdoctor.co.uk/womenshealth

NHS Direct www.nhsdirect.nhs.uk

Yoga

British Wheel of Yoga BWY Central Office, British Wheel of Yoga, 25 Jermyn Street, Sleaford, Lincolnshire NG34 7RU; Phone: 01529 306851; Web site: www.bwy.org.uk

Index

• _Q_ •

• _R_ •

Notes

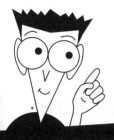

FOR DUMMIES®

Do Anything. Just Add Dummies

UK editions

PROPERTY

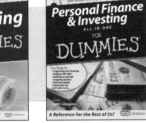

Buying and Selling a Home For Dummies
978-0-7645-7027-8

Renting Out Your Property For Dummies
978-0-470-02921-3

Buying a Property in Eastern Europe For Dummies
978-0-7645-7047-6

PERSONAL FINANCE

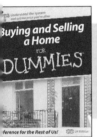

Investing For Dummies
978-0-7645-7023-0

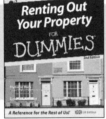

Personal Finance & Investing All-In-One For Dummies
978-0-470-51510-5

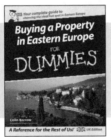

Bookkeeping For Dummies
978-0-470-05815-2

BUSINESS

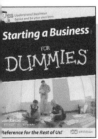

Starting a Business For Dummies
978-0-7645-7018-6

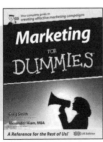

Marketing For Dummies
978-0-7645-7056-8

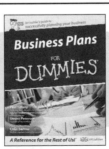

Business Plans For Dummies
978-0-7645-7026-1

Answering Tough Interview Questions For Dummies
(978-0-470-01903-0)

Arthritis For Dummies
(978-0-470-02582-6)

Being the Best Man For Dummies
(978-0-470-02657-1)

British History For Dummies
(978-0-470-03536-8)

Building Self-Confidence For Dummies
(978-0-470-01669-5)

Buying a Home on a Budget For Dummies
(978-0-7645-7035-3)

Children's Health For Dummies
(978-0-470-02735-6)

Cognitive Behavioural Therapy For Dummies
(978-0-470-01838-5)

Cricket For Dummies
(978-0-470-03454-5)

CVs For Dummies
(978-0-7645-7017-9)

Detox For Dummies
(978-0-470-01908-5)

Diabetes For Dummies
(978-0-470-05810-7)

Divorce For Dummies
(978-0-7645-7030-8)

DJing For Dummies
(978-0-470-03275-6)

eBay.co.uk For Dummies
(978-0-7645-7059-9)

English Grammar For Dummies
(978-0-470-05752-0)

Gardening For Dummies
(978-0-470-01843-9)

Genealogy Online For Dummies
(978-0-7645-7061-2)

Green Living For Dummies
(978-0-470-06038-4)

Hypnotherapy For Dummies
(978-0-470-01930-6)

Life Coaching For Dummies
(978-0-470-03135-3)

Neuro-linguistic Programming For Dummies
(978-0-7645-7028-5)

Nutrition For Dummies
(978-0-7645-7058-2)

Parenting For Dummies
(978-0-470-02714-1)

Pregnancy For Dummies
(978-0-7645-7042-1)

Rugby Union For Dummies
(978-0-470-03537-5)

Self Build and Renovation For Dummies
(978-0-470-02586-4)

Starting a Business on eBay.co.uk For Dummies
(978-0-470-02666-3)

Starting and Running an Online Business For Dummies
(978-0-470-05768-1)

The GL Diet For Dummies
(978-0-470-02753-0)

The Romans For Dummies
(978-0-470-03077-6)

Thyroid For Dummies
(978-0-470-03172-8)

UK Law and Your Rights For Dummies
(978-0-470-02796-7)

Writing a Novel and Getting Published For Dummies
(978-0-470-05910-4)

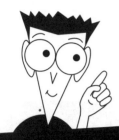

FOR DUMMIES®

Do Anything. Just Add Dummies

HOBBIES

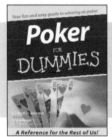

978-0-7645-5232-8

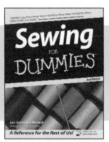

978-0-7645-6847-3

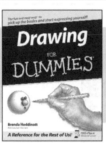

978-0-7645-5476-6

Also available:

Art For Dummies
(978-0-7645-5104-8)

Aromatherapy For Dummies
(978-0-7645-5171-0)

Bridge For Dummies
(978-0-471-92426-5)

Card Games For Dummies
(978-0-7645-9910-1)

Chess For Dummies
(978-0-7645-8404-6)

Improving Your Memory
For Dummies
(978-0-7645-5435-3)

Massage For Dummies
(978-0-7645-5172-7)

Meditation For Dummies
(978-0-471-77774-8)

Photography For Dummie
(978-0-7645-4116-2)

Quilting For Dummies
(978-0-7645-9799-2)

EDUCATION

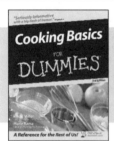

978-0-7645-7206-7

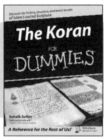

978-0-7645-5581-7

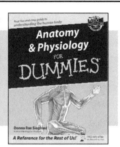

978-0-7645-5422-3

Also available:

Algebra For Dummies
(978-0-7645-5325-7)

Algebra II For Dummies
(978-0-471-77581-2)

Astronomy For Dummies
(978-0-7645-8465-7)

Buddhism For Dummies
(978-0-7645-5359-2)

Calculus For Dummies
(978-0-7645-2498-1)

Forensics For Dummies
(978-0-7645-5580-0)

Islam For Dummies
(978-0-7645-5503-9)

Philosophy For Dummies
(978-0-7645-5153-6)

Religion For Dummies
(978-0-7645-5264-9)

Trigonometry For Dummi
(978-0-7645-6903-6)

PETS

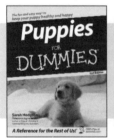

978-0-470-03717-1

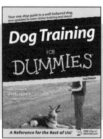

978-0-7645-8418-3

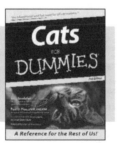

978-0-7645-5275-5

Also available:

Labrador Retrievers
For Dummies
(978-0-7645-5281-6)

Aquariums For Dummies
(978-0-7645-5156-7)

Birds For Dummies
(978-0-7645-5139-0)

Dogs For Dummies
(978-0-7645-5274-8)

Ferrets For Dummies
(978-0-7645-5259-5)

Golden Retrievers
For Dummies
(978-0-7645-5267-0)

Horses For Dummies
(978-0-7645-9797-8)

Jack Russell Terriers
For Dummies
(978-0-7645-5268-7)

Puppies Raising & Trainin
Diary For Dummies
(978-0-7645-0876-9)

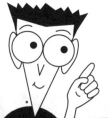

FOR DUMMIES®

The easy way to get more done and have more fun

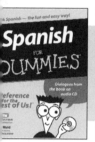
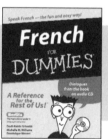
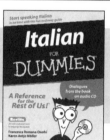
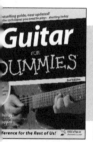
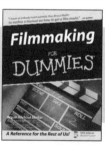
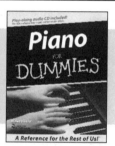
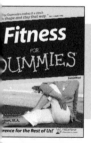
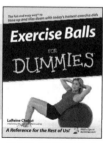
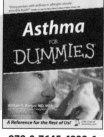

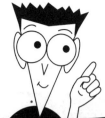

FOR DUMMIES®

Helping you expand your horizons and achieve your potenti[al]

INTERNET

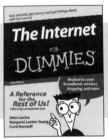

978-0-7645-8996-6

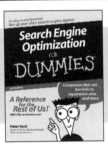

978-0-471-97998-2

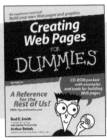

978-0-470-08030-6

Also available:

Building a Web Site For Dummies, 2nd Edition (978-0-7645-7144-2)

Blogging For Dummies For Dummies (978-0-471-77084-8)

eBay.co.uk For Dummies (978-0-7645-7059-9)

Web Analysis For Dummies (978-0-470-09824-0)

Web Design For Dummi[es] 2nd Edition (978-0-471-78117-2)

Creating Web Pages All-One Desk Reference For Dummies, 3rd Edition (978-0-470-09629-1)

DIGITAL MEDIA

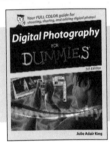

978-0-7645-9802-9

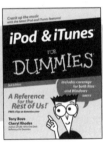

978-0-470-04894-8

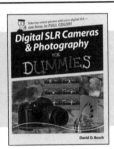

978-0-7645-9803-6

Also available:

Photoshop CS3 For Dummies (978-0-470-11193-2)

Podcasting For Dummies (978-0-471-74898-4)

Digital Photography All-In-One Desk Reference For Dummies (978-0-470-03743-0)

Digital Photo Projects For Dummies (978-0-470-12101-6)

BlackBerry For Dummie[s] (978-0-471-75741-2)

Zune For Dummies (978-0-470-12045-3)

COMPUTER BASICS

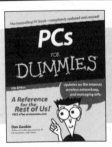

978-0-7645-8958-4

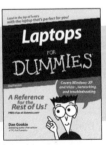

978-0-470-05432-1

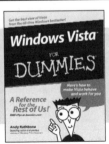

978-0-471-75421-3

Also available:

Macs For Dummies, 9th Edition (978-0-470-04849-8)

Windows Vista All-in-One Desk Reference For Dummies (978-0-471-74941-7)

Office 2007 All-in-One Desk Reference For Dummies (978-0-471-78279-7)

Windows XP For Dumm[ies] 2nd Edition (978-0-7645-7326-2)

PCs All-in-One Desk Re[fer]ence For Dummies, 3r[d Edi]tion (978-0-471-77082-4)

Upgrading & Fixing PC[s For] Dummies, 7th Edition (978-0-470-12102-3)
